YOUR FERTILITY PROGRAM

The East/West Guide to Maximum Fertility

Le

Bai
Dubi

Dr. Maureen Rozenn

This book is dedicated to my teachers, my mentors, and my patients.

༄

Contents

Introduction

Integrative Medicine in Practice - A Typical Day in the Gynecology/Fertility Department at the Second Affiliated Hospital of Zhejiang Chinese Medical University, Huang Zhou, China.

Mei Li patiently waited her turn to see Dr. Qin, the renowned fertility expert at Zhejiang Chinese Medical Hospital. She got there early enough, but even though she arrived well before Dr. Qin started seeing patients, there were dozens of women in front of her. They sat in chairs lining the hallway to Dr. Qin's office. Hours passed as she slowly inched closer to the office door. Hopefully, she could make it in before lunch. Finally she entered Dr. Qin's office and stood, along with several other women. The small room only had space for a desk and a few wooden chairs reserved for the doctor, her current patient, a translator and us: American Doctoral Candidates studying Chinese medical fertility treatment.

We sat in awe, hour after hour, as patient after patient filed in. Each brought their medical records with them. There was no privacy. Patients spoke freely of their diarrhea, the quality of their last menstrual period and the results of their medical tests. No one seemed bothered by this communal environment. It was drastically different than the health care model we are accustomed to in the United States, where patient privacy is highly valued. There were several other differences in the way health care was administered. Since patients keep their own charts, there are never problems communicating between doctors or instances of laboratory tests getting lost. A patient may have to wait several hours for the initial physician consultation, but after that she could get a physical exam, requisition for blood work, ultrasound or other imaging tests *and* discuss the results with her doctor ON THE SAME DAY! No spending weeks waiting for referrals to other specialists and no third party insurance agencies to approve tests, exams and treatments.

Mei Li was pleased to find herself in a chair opposite Dr. Qin well before lunch. Like all of the women preceding her, she handed Dr. Qin her last basal body temperature chart (BBT) and medical records. A 26 year old woman, Mei Li had been trying to conceive for 1 year. After reviewing her records and studying the BBT chart for a moment, Dr. Qin looked at Mei Li's tongue, felt her pulse and asked her several questions regarding sleep, digestion, ovulatory pain (middlesmirtz), energy, diet and exercise. Today was the 21st day of Mei Li's menstrual cycle. After carefully considering all of the information, Dr. Qin gave her a laboratory requisition for the hormone progesterone, as it was unclear from her BBT chart if she had ovulated. Mei Li thanked her physician and headed towards the laboratory.

After lunch, Mei Li walked back into Dr. Qin's office, ahead of other patients waiting in line for their first consult of the day. They sat down to discuss the results of her progesterone test. Mei Li's progesterone level was high enough to imply that she had ovulated this cycle, but it was not as high as Dr. Qin would have liked. She immediately typed Mei Li's herbal prescription into her computer, which links directly with the massive herbal pharmacy on the first floor of the hospital. Fourteen herbs were chosen for their ability to warm the womb, hold a pregnancy (if Mei Li was indeed pregnant), gently promote circulation to the reproductive organs, and strengthen the kidney yang. The prescription was geared to increase Mei Li's progesterone level as well.

Dr. Qin printed out a paper copy of the herbal prescription for Mei Li to keep in her medical file. Mei Li gladly headed downstairs to pick up her formula. She was instructed to return in ten days. If her period came and she was not pregnant, she would receive a new formula to enhance egg maturation and support uterine lining growth. If her period had not arrived, she would take a pregnancy test and receive herbal medicinals to either facilitate menstruation or to support her pregnancy.

After eight hours of watching Dr. Qin treat as many patients as I see in one week, I stepped out of the hospital into the scorching Southern China heat. I was overwhelmed by the breadth of information I had accumulated that day, as well as inspired to bring this experience and knowledge to my patients back home in the United States.

My Integrative Medicine Practice

I was a licensed acupuncturist for several years before going to China in 2009. The five weeks I spent studying fertility and gynecology in China was part of my Doctor of Acupuncture and Oriental Medicine (DAOM) curriculum. When Five Branches University announced that it would offer a DAOM program with specializations in Women's Health and Pain Management, I jumped to be in the first class. While a Master's in Traditional Chinese Medicine is the entry level degree for acupuncturists in California, I wanted to delve deeper into Classical Chinese texts, learn more acupuncture techniques and expand my repertoire of herbal formulas. In addition to numerous renowned Chinese medicine practitioners from the United States and China, my doctoral program included several classes in Western medicine taught by experts from Stanford University.

I spent six days per week at different affiliated Chinese medical hospitals and explored the rich history and beauty of China in my free time. I returned to the United States with innovative acupuncture methods and herbal prescriptions. More importantly, I gained a greater understanding of how integrative medicine could be practiced and applied to Women's Health and Fertility Treatment.

During my time in China I saw how Western laboratory tests, ultrasounds, acupuncture, and herbal prescriptions could be combined into a patient-based health care system. This was transformative for me. While I had practiced Integrative Medicine for years, witnessing how this East/West model worked seamlessly in Chinese hospitals was amazing.

It was at that point that I decided I wanted to go beyond specializing in Women's Health. I decided to do my doctoral thesis and attain board certification in Oriental Reproductive Medicine.

Since that time, I've been the lead acupuncturist and author on several research projects involving acupuncture and infertility. Two of these studies looked at specific acupuncture protocols pre and post in vitro fertilization (IVF) procedures. Another project examined an innovative method of treating unexplained infertility using both acupuncture and Clomid (a drug used to induce ovulation). Additionally, I co-wrote a study examining the effects of the Cridennda-Magarelli Acupuncture Protocol (CMAP) on the follicular fluid hormone levels of patients undergoing IVF. All of these studies were devised and implemented in conjunction with Western reproductive endocrinologists.

Through Five Branches and Yo San Universities, I have taught in both a Masters program in Traditional Chinese Medicine (MTCM) and in DAOM programs specializing in Oriental Reproductive Medicine. Students of all levels, from beginners to licensed acupuncturists, assist me in my clinic. I've spent as many years as an apprentice with different teachers as I've formally studied Integrative Medicine. Therefore, it is as important to me to keep the apprenticeship tradition alive, as it is to be a professor.

A fellow of the American Board of Oriental Reproductive Medicine (ABORM) and a California State licensed acupuncturist, I have a private practice focusing on Women's Health and Fertility Enhancement for men and women in Santa Cruz,

California. Research, teaching, and writing are my other passions, which led me to write this book.

The Book

Helping people make changes in their health and their lives is deeply rewarding to me. My patients are like my students. Yes, I am a doctor, but more importantly, I see myself as an educator. I teach people about their health: constitutional strengths and weaknesses, how the decisions they make in their everyday lives affect their health, and how to interpret their body's feedback. I endevor to empower my patients to make better choices and reach their health goals.

An ancient Taoist perspective holds that the secret to enhancing fertility is the same as engendering your own health and vitality. By living a healthier life, you slow the aging process and/or improve your potential to bring another life into this world. In essence, the goal is to help you become as healthy and strong as possible, then use that energy to enrich your own life and/or have a child.

What many people don't realize is that the state of their health before pregnancy can have a lasting impact on the vitality of their child, not to mention the quality of care they are able to provide the child directly after its birth. Parents need A LOT of energy to care for an infant. Too often we focus on the short-term goal of attaining pregnancy, but as you will learn, this is only part of the journey.

This book is written in a conversational format, mirroring the design of one of the oldest books on acupuncture and Chinese medical theory, the *Yellow Emperor's Inner Classic*. Legend has it that this text originated over four thousand years ago. It describes a conversation between the Yellow Emperor and his ministers on the nature of life, health, and our relationship to the universe. I figured that if a question and answer arrangement was good enough for the Yellow Emperor, it was good enough for us.

As this is an Integrative Medicine book, we will be talking about both Eastern and Western concepts of organ function. For clarity, I've capitalized organ names when I'm discussing them in an Oriental Medical (OM) context. When I'm referring to their Western medical functions the organ names are not capitalized. Additionally, I've included some of my patients' stories and several research studies that are based on sound science.

As acupuncture and OM are new to me, can you tell me what happens during the first visit?

Good question! The initial consultation begins with a thorough medical intake. A well-trained practitioner should ask you about your family medical history, important milestones in your life, sleep, digestion, energy, musculoskeletal system, emotional patterns and immune system, before even getting to your reproductive system! We ask women about their menstrual cycles and gynecological history. We may order blood tests to check pituitary, ovarian function and/or recommend other means of mapping the menstrual cycle and determining the time of ovulation, such as: BBT charting, the OV-watch or LH surge predictor tests.

In addition to taking your medical history and reviewing any prior laboratory reports and herbal, nutraceutical or pharmacological substances you are currently taking, I also conduct a physical examination consisting of tongue, pulse and abdominal diagnosis. Only after all of these steps are taken do I perform an acupuncture treatment. The acupuncture point prescription is unique to each patient and is determined by the individual's OM diagnosis. Oriental Medicine is based in ancient Chinese medicine but is much broader, encompassing diagnostics, theories, and therapeutic techniques developed in Japan, Korea and other Asian countries. A very important aspect of OM is that each patient be individually diagnosed and treated. Ten women with the Western label of endometriosis might each receive a different OM diagnosis and thus be prescribed different herbal medicinals, acupuncture points and nutraceuticals.

Fertility protocols for women generally focus on promoting egg development, uterine lining enhancement, and regulation of the endocrine system. Treatment for men centers on improved circulation to the reproductive organs to enhance sexual vitality and semen quality. Detoxification and antioxidants are key aspects to fertility promotion for both sexes.

The Modalities of Oriental Medicine

Once a diagnosis has been made, practitioners have a variety of techniques to choose from to correct imbalances. While acupuncture is the most well known OM modality, other useful tools include moxabustion and herbal therapy.

Acupuncture dates back over 2,000 years. Acupuncture regulates qi to stimulate the body's own healing process. "Qi" roughly translates to "vital energy". We will talk more about qi in following chapters. Acupuncture treatments consist of placing thin, sterile, disposable needles in specific areas of the body called acupuncture points. These points are located on meridians, which are pathways in the body that carry qi. The meridian system is analogous to the circulatory system, where blood vessels transport blood, and the nervous system, where nerves carry nerve impulses. Every organ has a meridian that runs between that organ and the surface of the body. Sometimes qi becomes blocked in a meridian, which can disrupt blood flow causing changes in organ function and/or pain along the meridian. Late ovulation, irregular menstrual cycles, PMS and menstrual cramps can all be caused by blocked qi. There are many reasons why qi becomes blocked, such as poor dietary habits, stress, lack of exercise, physical and emotional trauma, overexertion, infections, seasonal changes or a weak constitution. By stimulating points on specific meridians, practitioners can unblock qi and stimulate blood flow, thereby regulating the menstrual cycle and promoting fertility.

Moxabustion is not as well known, but it is just as important as acupuncture. The Chinese word for acupuncture is more accurately translated as "acumoxa". For hundreds of years acupuncture and moxabustion have been used together in clinical practice to prevent and treat illness. Moxabustion consists of gently warming acupuncture points with moxa (dried mugwort). It is used to improve digestion, regulate menstruation, stimulate ovulation, reduce menstrual cramps, and stop excessive menstrual bleeding.

Herbology in China has evolved through centuries of carefully documented clinical experience. Through this process, extensive information has been gathered detailing not only the properties of single herbs, but also how herbs interact in formulas. Today, we have the benefit of combining this empirical data (data derived from clinical or practical experience) with several different types of scientific studies. A variety of research reports have given us insight into the chemical composition of individual herbs, while large-scale trials conducted in China and Japan yield data on the use of herbal formulas for modern-day conditions.

Recently, there have been concerns raised about the purity of individual Chinese herbs and ready-made formulas in terms of their pharmaceutical, heavy metal and pesticide content. Reputable manufacturers of herbal formulas in China, Japan and the United States routinely test their herbs for pesticides, fumigants and bacteria, and reject shipments that fail to meet their strict standards. Though most prepared Chinese herbal formulas are safe, without harmful pesticides, heavy metals or pharmaceuticals, one should only take herbal preparations when prescribed by a trained health care professional.

I could try herbs, even moxabustion, but I'm afraid of needles.

This is a common concern. Acupuncture is relatively new to the West. When people think of needles they remember childhood traumas, shots and giving blood. Those procedures are done with hollow needles. Unlike those hypodermic needles, the needles used for acupuncture are about the width of a hair. You may feel a little poke or pinch, upon the initial insertion, but the sensation from an acupuncture needle should be very mild. Treatments last for about 25 minutes. Acupuncture is very relaxing for most people. Many patients even nap during treatment!

After the acupuncture treatment, the initial visit concludes with a comprehensive fertility enhancement plan. The plan outlines steps to correct not only symptoms (such as irregular and painful menstruation, lack of ovulation and low sperm counts), but also the underlying causes of infertility: yin deficiency, yang deficiency or qi/blood stagnation. We will talk about what each of these terms mean in detail in the following chapters.

Research on OM Fertility Treatment

Given Oriental Medicine's long history of treating gynecological problems and infertility, it's not surprising that one of the most popular areas of international acupuncture research today is the field of fertility enhancement. Studies done in China, Germany, Italy, the United States and Sweden have demonstrated that acupuncture and herbal formulas can regulate the menstrual cycle, induce ovulation, and augment Western Assisted Reproductive Therapies (ART). Additionally, there have been several studies showing that OM can improve male fertility. Semen parameters, such as sperm motility, morphology, and quality can be improved with OM. We will talk specifically about research studies and male fertility in chapter 5. Currently, there are a handful of fertility clinics in the United States conducting research on the use of OM modalities for both male and female fertility enhancement.

Empirical evidence shows that OM can regulate menstruation and support fertility. There is also a significant pile of evidence demonstratrating higher successful in vitro fertilization (IVF) outcomes when acupuncture treatments are added to the treatment protocol. Additionally, acupuncture has been shown to positively effect uterine blood flow, the neuroendocrine system, hypothalamic-pituitary-ovarian axis, and ovulation.

OM excels in some areas of fertility for which Western medicine has no treatment. One such area is endometrial thickness. Embryos need a soft, plush uterine lining to burrow into. A frequently cited study by Sterner-Victorin et al. shows that acupuncture can increase blood flow to the uterus and endometrium. The authors of the study believe this effect is accomplished through acupuncture's calming affect on the nervous system. Their deduction is supported by several research studies on depression, anxiety and stress, demonstrating that acupuncture affects endorphin levels in addition to regulating the nervous system.

Acupuncture has been used since the 1960's in rural hospitals in China to induce ovulation. At that time, the reported success rate was as high as 50%. Since that time, numerous studies have demonstrated OM's ability to induce ovulation, increase the size of ovarian follicles and estrogen, follicle stimulating hormone (FSH) and luteinizing hormone (LH) levels.

On the whole, research shows that OM can increase live birth rates, reduce birth complications and improve IVF outcomes. This area is rife for further study. In 2010, I co-wrote a research study examining the effect of a specific acupuncture protocol and IVF outcomes, because I believe it is crucial that we conduct well-designed research studies in this area.

It is my intention that you use this book as a guide on your journey to improved health, fertility, and healthy babies. Feel free to flip through the following chapters and focus on what is relevant to you. This East/West guide to boosting fertility covers the most commonly asked questions and concerns about Oriental and Western reproductive enhancement techniques. Use the information presented in the following chapters as a comprehensive guide to better health and family building!

Yours in health,

Dr. Maureen Rozenn, LAC, DAOM, FABORM

The Roots of Fertility

CHINESE MEDICINE HAS THE longest recorded history of any medical system, with a rich tradition of treating gynecological problems and promoting fertility. Ancient writings found on bones and shells describe strategies for treating difficulties during childbirth. Other texts on the use of herbal medicinals for infertility were written over 2000 years ago.

The *Yellow Emperor's Inner Classic* is one of the oldest surviving Chinese medical manuscripts. This book dates back to 2600 BCE. It sets forth the foundations of modern Oriental Medical (OM) theory and contains extensive passages on the physiology and pathophysiology of menstruation, fertility and pregnancy. From a woman's first period (menarche) until her last (menopause), the ancient Chinese described in detail the hormonal changes that take place throughout a woman's lifetime and the factors that influence this process.

While each organ system has an important role in menstruation, fertility and pregnancy, the Heart and the Kidneys have a special relationship with the Uterus. The Chinese use the word "Uterus" to represent a number of endocrine organs and structures such as the ovaries, fallopian tubes, pituitary and hypothalamus.

Heaven & Earth/Nature & Nurture

Long before we in the West started unraveling the mysteries of DNA, the Chinese had fully integrated the concept of genetics (referred to as pre-heaven essence or "jing") into their medical theory. Jing is the substance we received from our parents and is stored in the Kidneys. It is the foundation of our constitution, our genetic tendencies and forms the basis of what we will pass on to our offspring. Ovarian follicles are an expression of jing. Women are born with all of their ovarian follicles, which have the potential to become eggs. The number and quality of these follicles is dependent on the strength of their Kidneys and jing.

So, I was born with all the eggs I will ever have? I can't make more?

Correct. They were actually formed with your organs during your development in your mother's uterus.

The fact that we have two Kidneys is significant in Chinese philosophy and medicine. The Kidneys are the source of all of our yin and yang. Yin and yang are metaphors used in Chinese philosophy/medicine that represent opposing forces. Yin is the cool, dark, moist, creative force, in contrast to yang, which is bright, forceful, and uplifting. We can see these forces at play in the world: a lake is yin, a desert is yang, day is yang, night is yin, summer is yang, winter is yin and so on. A cornerstone belief of OM is that the human body is a microcosm of the universe. Thus, the forces that govern the world also influence us. We go through cycles of yin and yang just like the seasons change. The Kidney organ system is responsible for guiding us through hormonal changes during our lifetime as well as supporting the hormonal shifts (yin shifting to yang) in a single menstrual cycle. We need adequate amounts of yin and yang to have a healthy menstrual cycle, conception, and pregnancy.

We know genetics isn't everything. Just because something "runs in the family" doesn't mean we have to succumb to it. For example, one may have a genetic tendency towards high blood pressure because both parents have it, but that doesn't mean that person is destined to develop high blood pressure. The lifestyle and dietary choices you make every day can dramatically influence your health and which genetic tendencies you express.

Just as the Kidneys are the source of pre-heaven essence, the Spleen, Stomach and Pancreas (collectively referred to as the "Spleen" in OM theory) are the source of post-heaven essence. The Spleen is directly responsible for assimilating nutrients from food and transforming them into blood, body fluids and qi. While blood cells are made in the bone marrow, according to the Chinese, the digestive system is equally important in determining an individual's quality and quantity of blood.

I thought the spleen was part of the immune system.

In Western medical theory that is correct. The spleen functions somewhat like a giant lymph node, filtering the blood. In OM, the Spleen plays a part in immune function. Interestingly, it also plays a pivotal role in OM because the Spleen is instrumental in making the essential substances: qi, blood and body fluids.

Tears and synovial fluid (responsible for joint lubrication) are examples of body fluids. Their job is to keep tissues moist. Cervical mucus is a type of body fluid that changes during ovulation to assist the sperm in their journey towards the fallopian tubes and hopefully an oocyte. Healthy body fluids have an appropriate consistency —not too thin or too thick. Body fluids that are too thick are classified as phlegm.

Qi

Qi is not a concept we have in Western medicine. Unlike blood and body fluids, it cannot be seen with the naked eye. Qi roughly translates to "vital energy". Every living thing in the universe has qi coursing through it. Qi is what animates us; it is the spark of life that makes us different from inanimate objects. Qi innervates every muscle, organ, and fiber of our bodies. Every action we take, including talking, reading, and thinking, all require the movement of qi.

The body needs high quality, abundant blood, qi and body fluids to ovulate, form a thick, healthy uterine lining and sustain a pregnancy. For example, if phlegm occurs from faulty body fluid metabolism, it can block the fallopian tubes or in the case of Polycystic Ovarian Syndrome (PCOS), inhibit ovulation.

My aunt lived to be 99 and ate nothing but bacon, eggs and steak. She had coffee every day and could drink anyone under the table, except me. Does that mean I can live this way and have 8 children?

The state of our health is a complex interplay between pre and post-heaven essence. Some people are born with very strong pre-heaven essence. These are the people who smoke, drink, eat sugary, greasy foods and live over a hundred years. Most of us, however, are not that sturdy. There is significant debate within the OM community on the potential of adding to one's pre-heaven essence. What is agreed upon, is that while the aging process depletes jing, you can conserve and nourish it by making the most of your post-heaven essence. Eating well and living a healthy lifestyle are two of the most important things you can do to augment your post-heaven essence, preserve your jing, and enhance fertility.

Your body wants to conceive; this is a natural process, which can be helped tremendously with just a few nudges in the right direction.

The Will of Reproduction

The Kidneys are associated with willpower in Chinese medical theory. Connected to the Uterus through the Bao Luo (uterus circulation), the Kidneys rule this meridian. Through this relationship, the Uterus receives pre-heaven energy and the will to procreate.

The Kidneys endow the uterine lining (endometrium) with the potential to nourish new life and support healthy egg (follicle) maturation and ovulation. Should a pregnancy occur, it is the Kidneys that give the Uterus strength to secure the pregnancy. If a woman suffers from a weak Kidney organ system, she may have irregular menstruation or menstrual cycles without ovulating (anovulatory cycles) and be prone to miscarriages.

I have had 2 miscarriages. Does that mean there is something wrong with my kidneys?

No. The Western view of kidney function and the OM definition of Kidney health are two very different concepts. While a urinalysis or blood test are used to determine kidney function, in OM theory, women who have had more than one miscarriage almost universally need to strengthen their Kidneys.

The Uterus-A Woman's Second Heart

Every woman is aware (as are most men, if they know what's good for them), that emotional states are tied to hormonal fluctuations. A familiar description of this phenomenon is Premenstrual Syndrome (PMS). First documented by Western scientists in the 1930's, PMS is a complex syndrome encompassing hundreds of possible physical and psychological symptoms. These can occur anywhere from two weeks to just a few hours prior to the onset of menses. Common symptoms include: irritability, headaches, depression, bloating, food cravings, breast tenderness, anxiety, and mood swings. While up to 40% of menstruating women experience moderate to severe PMS, it is estimated that 5% of women have Premenstrual Dysphoric Disorder (PMDD), an extremely severe and debilitating form of PMS in which behavioral and emotional symptoms predominate. PMS can have dramatic social and economic ramifications for these women, resulting in loss of income and interpersonal relationship problems. Common Western treatments for these issues are comprised of the birth control pill and antidepressants. They are geared towards reducing symptoms through hormonal and brain chemistry stabilization.

While we in the West are just starting to understand the relationship between moods and hormonal shifts, these concepts were outlined in Chinese medical texts thousands of years ago. Ancient manuscripts describe the connection between emotional states and hormonal balance as the relationship between the Heart and the Uterus. Rather than the brain being the organ that determines behavior, in Classic Chinese medical theory, this is the Heart's domain.

The written Chinese language is comprised of characters, which are essentially simplified pictures. The characters for the Heart protector (Pericardium) and the Uterus are almost identical. The difference is that the character for Uterus encompasses the picture for "flesh". As the Heart pumps blood, the Uterus also cyclically fills and empties with blood. The Pericardium protects the Heart so that it can rhythmically beat, representing the surging of life, while the Uterus is where life grows and is protected. Thus, the Uterus functions as a woman's second Heart.

Just as the Kidneys and the Uterus connect through the Bao Luo, the Heart and the Uterus communicate with each other via the Bao Mai, which literally translates to "Uterus Vessel". Every month, blood comes down from the Heart through the Bao Mai and settles in the Uterus, providing the Uterus with the potential to nourish an embryo. The Bao Mai must be open and unimpeded for menstruation and conception to occur. If this link is disrupted, women can experience PMS symptoms in addition to irregular menstrual cycles and infertility.

How does this disruption occur?

Stress and emotional upheavals are both the cause and effect of a blockage in the Bao Mai.

Bao Mai, is that like an artery or nerve? I don't understand.

Neither. It is a passageway that allows qi and blood to flow directly between the Heart and Uterus. When we look at this intuitively, it makes sense. Most women have experienced the consequences of a Bao Mai blockage. For example, almost universally, women find their PMS gets worse in times of increased stress and psychological pressure. Also, many women have had the experience of missing a period due to emotional duress.

The wisdom of OM tells us that both the Heart and the Uterus are intimately connected and that the healthy functioning of one depends on the other.

Reading Your Body's Fertility Signals

SUSAN, AN INTELLIGENT, YOUNG looking 40 year old, first came to see me with a simple question, "Am I healthy enough to get pregnant?" This is a simple question with a complicated answer. I was the first physician she had seen in search of the answer.

"Well", I said, "let's see if we can answer that question". I began by asking about her general health, including her menstrual cycle and prior pregnancies. Then I asked her some very basic questions regarding her fertility, starting with, "Do you ovulate on your own, and if so, on what day of your cycle?".

She had no idea. I asked if she had ever used Luteinizing Hormone surge detectors, the OV-Watch, temperature charting, or other Fertility Awareness Methods. She had not. Finding out if Susan was ovulating was the first step in answering her question. Obviously, no ovulation equals no pregnancy.

Susan is not alone. Many women are mystified by their menstrual cycle and have no idea when they are fertile. They don't know that there are ways to answer these questions on their own. In this chapter, we're going to talk about how you can get some of your own answers through a variety of self-observation techniques.

The Menstrual Cycle, Yawn

I don't know about you, but when I was in high school nothing would put me to sleep faster than trying to memorize the series of hormonal fluctuations in the menstrual cycle. In college, my boredom turned to mixed interest and confusion as I tried to piece together the complex interconnected feedback loops of the neuro-endocrine system. Now, I am in a state of utter fascination and awe as I look at women's reproductive cycles, not just in a Western sense, but from an OM perspective as well.

We could take several hundred pages to explain all of the inner workings of the hypothalamus-pituitary-ovarian axis. Hundreds more pages could be filled describing how it is influenced by the autonomic nervous system, thyroid and adrenals (a.k.a. jing, Kidney and Spleen organ systems, qi, blood, yin and yang). But, let's not. For our purposes, we will keep it simple and practical. Understanding the basics of the menstrual cycle is the first step towards gaining control over your fertility.

The Basics: East/West

Most women have approximately a 28-day menstrual cycle. The cycle begins with the first day of menstrual bleeding. In Western medicine, the cycle is divided into two phases, the follicular phase and the luteal phase. Now don't go to sleep yet! Basically, during the first part of your cycle (follicular phase), estrogen levels increase, causing ovarian follicles to develop and mature. Eventually, one follicle becomes the biggest, most dominate follicle and the other follicles wither away. This follicle is now ready to be released from the ovary (ovulation). This act marks the second part of your cycle (luteal phase). After the egg (oocyte) pops out of the ovary, it makes it way down the fallopian tube. The fallopian tubes are structures that connect your ovaries to your uterus. Ideally, the sperm meet the oocyte in the fallopian tube. Thus, fertilization takes place before the oocyte gets to the uterus. These tubes must be open and flexible for the sperm and oocyte to unite and be guided to the uterus.

During the luteal phase, progesterone levels rise. Should an embryo implant in the lining of the uterus (endometrium), high levels of progesterone keep the embryo in place and prevent menstruation. If there is no embryo, your progesterone levels drop, you start your period and the process begins all over again.

In OM, the menstrual cycle is divided into yin (follicular) and yang (luteal) phases. During the yin phase, we want to nourish yin and blood to assist in the production of healthy, mature follicles and a thick endometrium. When the egg is released from the ovary, the yang takes over. In the yang phase, it is crucial to support the yang and to gently promote blood circulation to the pelvic organs. This ensures that if an embryo is present, it can implant in the endometrium and the body can support the pregnancy, rather than releasing it with a period. Miscarriages can occur during this crucial time if there is not enough yang (progesterone) to prepare the uterus and hold the pregnancy.

A Little More Than the Basics—Western

Now that we have mastered the basics, lets go a little deeper. How does the ovary know when to release an egg? In fact, how does it know when to start maturing follicles so you have an egg to release at ovulation time? To answer these questions we have to talk about the pituitary gland.

The pituitary is a very interesting little part of the brain that guides the ovaries in maturing follicles and releasing eggs. It does this by sending hormones to the ovaries. Follicle Stimulating Hormone (FSH) is the hormone the pituitary sends to the ovaries to signal them to start maturing follicles. Luteinizing Hormone (LH) is the hormone the pituitary releases to signal the ovaries that it is time to release an egg (ovulate).

Now I suspect your ears are starting to perk up. If you have started the process of trying to conceive, you probably recognize the term LH. This hormone is easily tested, by urine strips available at your local pharmacy, to determine the time of ovulation. If the ovary reacts properly to the LH signal from the pituitary, an egg should be released within 24-48 hours. The catch is, those strips only measure the LH surge. They do not determine the health of the eggs and endometrium or if the ovary is going to respond appropriately to LH and actually ovulate.

What tells the pituitary what to do?

Yet another part of the brain, the hypothalamus. The hypothalamus monitors levels of various hormones and decides when to tell the pituitary to increase one hormone or decrease another.

What about the thyroid gland, doesn't it play a role in regular menstrual cycles and fertility?

Yes, absolutely. We will talk more about the thyroid in the Pregnancy and Fertility Challenges chapter.

How does stress affect fertility?

We will discuss this subject in-depth throughout this entire book. In brief, stress negatively impacts fertility in many ways. It activates the sympathetic or "fight or flight" aspect of the nervous system and shuts down the parasympathetic or "feed and breed" part of the nervous system. Through this action, it decreases pelvic circulation and specifically impacts blood flow to the uterus. Stress can cause numerous endocrine imbalances as well. Rather than having adequate levels of progesterone (the pro-gestation hormone), under stress, the body focuses on making more cortisol. This can be both the cause and effect of many endocrine and metabolic problems like Insulin Resistance Syndrome, Polycystic Ovary Disease, Recurrent Miscarriages and more…

But let's not get ahead of ourselves. We will talk about all of these issues in detail in the Pregnancy and Fertility Challenges and Diet & Lifestyle chapters. For now, let's turn our attention to learning what happens during a healthy menstrual cycle from an OM point of view.

A Little More Than the Basics—OM

Leading up to menstrual cycle day one, there should be very little PMS, as the Bao Mai is open and flowing smoothly. Ideally, bleeding should occur for 4-7 days with no clots or cramping. While most Western physicians consider between 21-35 days a normal cycle length, OM gynecologists prefer the menstrual cycle to be as close to 28 days as possible. Cycles that are too long or too short indicate a yin and yang imbalance, as it is the healthy interaction of these two forces that produces a fertile menstrual cycle.

Menstrual Cycle Phase One—Yin & Blood

On day one of the cycle, a dramatic shift occurs as yang reaches its height and becomes yin. In Western medicine we would say it is during this time that progesterone and estrogen levels fall and menses starts. While bleeding can last for seven days, (or longer in some women) generally by day 4, the uterine lining starts to rebuild itself. So, as we are cleaning out the old we are simultaneously building up the new endometrium and preparing for another potential pregnancy.

Under the dominance of yin, the lining of the uterus continues to grow and the ovarian follicles begin to mature. As these eggs mature, they secrete estrogen, which is regarded as a yin hormone. The endometrium responds to estrogen by increasing in size. Fertility specialists can augment this process through acupuncture and by prescribing blood and yin strengthening herbal formulas, thus enhancing endometrial thickness and egg development.

The Menstrual Cycle Phase Two—Yang & Qi

As the uterine lining becomes full and lush and the egg ripens, yin reaches its zenith and shifts to yang. Cervical fluid changes and the body prepares to ovulate. During ovulation the mature egg bursts forth from the follicle under the influence of qi. Remember, qi represents dynamic movement. It is this spark of qi that happens when yin shifts to yang, causing the ovary to release the egg. This spark is roughly equivalent to the Western concept of LH. During this crucial time in the cycle, the pituitary and ovary must work together to ensure that ovulation occurs. If the egg is released too early, it may not be fully developed, and if fertilized, the embryo is prone to chromosomal defects. Even if the embryo is perfectly healthy, the lining of the uterus may be too thin and insufficient to nourish the rapidly growing embryo.

Should ovulation occurs too late, we face the possibility of genetic defects and higher miscarriage rates. Emotional disturbances, which affect the Bao Mai, can disrupt the timing of ovulation, as can delayed egg development due to blood and yin deficiency. Herbal formulas and acupuncture are used mid-cycle to regulate this process. Herbs that move qi can help the egg break free. Also, through moving qi, acupuncture can induce ovulation and promote the smooth passage of the egg down the fallopian tube.

Acupuncture's Effect on the Hypothalamus, Pituitary and Ovaries

In 1997 Dr. Chen published an important piece of research, Acupuncture Normalizes Dysfunction of Hypothalamic-Pituitary-Ovarian Axis, in which he states that in China the success rate of acupuncture in inducing ovulation is 80%. He wanted to know why. In this landmark paper he discusses studies on both humans and animals showing that acupuncture can regulate the key fertility hormones such as estrogen and LH. He also showed that acupuncture could influence the nervous system, support hormonal balance and optimal reproductive functioning.

After ovulation, the follicle that once secreted estrogen becomes the corpus luteum and releases progesterone. Progesterone is regarded as a yang hormone. Progesterone causes your body temperature to rise slightly after ovulation. Your temperature should remain elevated throughout the luteal phase, not dropping again until the first day of your period. This heat dries up the cervical fluid, changing it from the fertile-moist-elastic fluid into a sticky substance, which actually acts as a barrier to the uterus. During the yang part of the cycle, progesterone warms the womb by causing the endometrium to produce nutrients in anticipation of pregnancy. If implantation occurs, the progesterone levels will continue to increase, maintaining this "progesterone fever".

So, after my temperature rises, my cervical fluid dries up and the sperm have a harder time even getting into the uterus. How am I supposed to get pregnant at this point?

The short answer is, you don't. Pregnancy is most likely to occur when intercourse takes place the day before or the day of ovulation. After your temperature rises you can hold off on actively trying to conceive for another month.

But how do I know what specific day(s) are the best for intercourse?

This is where the Fertility Awareness Method (FAM) comes into play. Now that you know the physiology behind your menstrual cycle, you can use FAM to pinpoint the best days for conception. We will discuss FAM in the next section of this chapter.

If the timing is right, the egg has properly developed and spit out of the ovary. Also, the sperm is well formed and able to fertilize the egg in the fallopian tube. Then, about four days after ovulation, the healthy embryo finds its way to the uterus. It will be about 8-10 days after ovulation when the uterine lining is at its greatest size and most receptive state. At this stage of the cycle, OM fertility specialists focus on warming the yang and maintaining high progesterone levels to enable the body to sustain the pregnancy. During this phase, acupuncture is used to gently promote the movement of qi, relax and nourish the womb, and reduce any PMS symptoms.

If implantation does not occur, because there was no union with a sperm, the embryo had chromosomal defects or the endometrium was not receptive, yang shifts back to yin and the process starts anew.

Fertility Awareness Method (FAM)

The Fertility Awareness Method (FAM) has its roots in the early 20th century. Efforts to improve the effectiveness of the Rhythm Method of birth control (the only birth control method approved by the Catholic Church) prompted research into the effect hormonal shifts have on women's basal temperatures. In the 1930's a German Catholic priest, Reverend Wilhelm Hillebrand, advocated using Basal Body Temperatures (BBT's) as an acceptable method of birth control. The goal was to determine when ovulation occurred in order to avoid conception. Later, in the 1950's, scientists discovered the relationship between changes in cervical fluid (CF) and the fertile peak in the menstrual cycle. Twenty years later, in the 1970s, the Couple to Couple League International group combined BBTs, with cervical position (CP) and fluid to create the Sympto-Thermal Method, also known as FAM.

The FAM is far more personalized and reliable than the Rhythm Method for family planning. The Rhythm Method assumes the all women ovulate on day 14 of their menstrual cycle and suggests avoiding (or engaging in, if pregnancy is desired) intercourse the week before ovulation. If used for contraceptive purposes, the Rhythm Method is approximately 13% effective, while FAM boasts a 99.5% success rate. This is nearly as effective as the birth control pill, which is estimated to be 99.8% effective.

It stands to reason that if a woman can collect information about her menstrual cycle in order to AVOID pregnancy, she can also use that data to BECOME pregnant. Therefore, the FAM can be used to increase the chances of pregnancy by determining fertile days and engaging in intercourse during that time.

Oriental Medicine has evolved through keen observation of both the universe at large and the human body. Throughout its long history of treating infertility, information such as the timing, duration and color of menses has been an integral part of diagnosis and assessing response to treatment. In modern times, OM gynecologists have integrated BBT charting into their diagnostic process.

During my studies at Zhejiang Chinese Medical Hospital, every woman seeking herbal treatment for infertility, endometriosis, PCOS and recurrent miscarriage brought their BBT chart to each appointment. The OM gynecologist incorporated the chart into traditional methods of diagnosis such as pulse and tongue readings. All of this information was used to form a diagnosis and formulate an herbal formula specific to the patient's condition and phase of her cycle.

Now, let's put all of the information we have learned about the phases of the menstrual cycle to good use. The more you know about your cycle, the better you are able to answer such questions as: Are you ovulating? If so, when? What is the strength of your follicular/yin and luteal/yang phases? These fertility awareness methods will help you pinpoint your fertile times and give you clues about any obstacles you may have to pregnancy.

Next we're going to discuss the three most important aspects of FAM, namely BBT, CP and CF.

Basal Body Temperature Charting (BBT)

BBT charting brings a woman in touch with her body's unique hormonal profile. Because key fertility hormones such as estrogen and progesterone affect the temperature-regulating center of the brain, we can infer hormonal patterns by measuring the basal (or baseline) temperature. Remember, estrogen is a yin, moist, cool hormone. Therefore, during the yin/follicular phase, temperatures should be lower than during the yang/luteal phase, in which warmer progesterone predominates. You should be able to see a distinct temperature shift that indicates ovulation. If this dramatic temperature change is not clear, the BBT pattern provides clues as to why you're not ovulating, or possibly what is hindering your fertility.

Getting Started

First you need to find a chart you like. There are several to choose from. Some include very basic information, while others have space to include detailed information such as headaches, breast soreness, moodiness, etc. The most important factors to track are: intercourse, days of bleeding, days of CF, the quality of the CF, CP, the results of LH surge predictor kits, your temperature and <u>WHAT TIME</u> in the morning you took your temperature. The time is critical because your temperature naturally rises as the morning progresses by about 0.2 degrees F per hour.

Many women like to keep a printed chart on their bedside table, but there are also electronic options for tracking fertility information. There are several applications for cell phones, numerous websites and software available where you can store the details of your menstrual cycle and chart your fertility. There are also have several thermometer choices. These vary from mercury to digital, Fahrenheit to Celsius. No matter what type of thermometer you choose, make sure it is accurate to one-tenth of a degree. Typically these thermometers will state clearly on the package that they are Basal Body Temperature Thermometers or intended for fertility charting. You can find these online and in most drug stores. No matter what kind of tracking devices you opt for, keep them by your bed so they are readily available when you wake up in the morning.

During the follicular phase, your temperatures should be lower than after ovulation. Typically, on <u>THE DAY OF</u> ovulation your temperature will dip even lower, and then shoot up over the next few days. This is the signal that yin has reached its zenith and turned to yang. In other words, ovulation has occurred and progesterone levels are rising.

Your temperature should stay elevated until progesterone and estrogen levels drop. At this point, your chart will show a dramatic temperature decrease signaling that your period is about to begin. If, after 18 days post ovulation, your temperature does not drop and you do not get your period, this could indicate that progesterone levels have remained elevated and pregnancy has occurred. It's time to take a pregnancy test!

How to Chart

Start recording your temperature on day 1 of your cycle (the first day of menstrual bleeding). For an accurate reading, the temperature should be taken at the same time every morning and after at least 3 (though 5 is preferable) hours of uninterrupted sleep. As soon as you wake up, before urinating, cuddling, drinking water, etc. take your temperature and record it on your graph.

I took my temperature for a month. How do I make sense out of my chart?

When evaluating the BBT for a full menstrual cycle, take the average follicular phase temperature and subtract it from the average luteal phase temperature. This is the overall temperature change between the two phases, which is called a "thermal shift". Ovulation and subsequent progesterone levels that are sufficient to maintain a pregnancy are reflected by a rise in temperature of at least .04 degrees, though .06 or more is preferable. Follicular phase temperatures are typically between 96.5 and 98.0, while luteal phase temperatures should range from about 97.7 and 99.0 degrees. The healthiest follicular phases are marked by relatively stable temperatures that don't fluctuate more than 0.3 degrees. The key indicator to look for in luteal phase temperatures is that the rise after ovulation is maintained for at least 12 days. Also, we don't want to see temperatures drop to pre-ovulation levels until menses occurs. A sharp decrease in temperature should indicate that menstruation is imminent.

What if my temperature does not drop? In fact, what if it rises even higher, to develop from a biphasic (two phase) into a triphasic (three phase) chart?

If you haven't already, it is definitely time to take a pregnancy test. Often in early pregnancy temperatures will rise even higher than during the luteal phase, instead of dropping with menstruation.

It is important to take your temperature as close to the same time as possible each morning. Your temperature will naturally be lower in the early morning and rise throughout the day. It is less important what time you take your temperature (i.e. either 6am or 9am) and more important that you take it at a consistent time. Illness, stress, alcohol intake, travel, late nights and restless sleep can raise your temperature and give you erroneous or misleading information about your hormone levels. Common non-steroidal anti-inflammatory drugs (NSAIDs) such as Tylenol or Motrin can lower your temperature. Mouth breathing can throw off a BBT chart. Women who snore may want to take their temperature vaginally or rectally. However, don't change the site where you take your temperature during a cycle. This should be taken into account when calculating your overall follicular and luteal phase temperatures.

Additional Factors That Can Alter BBT Charts

- Electric blankets
- Sleep-aid drugs
- Anti-anxiety medications (except benzodiazepines)
- Antihistamines, statins, anti-psychotics, anti-depressants (SSRIS and Tricyclics)

Cervical Position (CP)

Cervical position and secretions can tell you a lot about hormonal cycles and peak fertile days as both position and cervical fluid consistency change throughout the menstrual cycle.

To feel your cervix, wash your hands, keep your nails short and gently insert two fingers into your vagina. Carefully feel your CP and texture. During menses and shortly afterwards, the cervix is in a low position, meaning that you can easily reach it with your fingers. Notice also that the texture of the cervix is hard and the opening is relatively small and tight. All of these signs indicate that this is not a fertile time in your cycle.

Shortly before ovulation the cervix will start to rise, reaching its highest point at ovulation. At this time, the surface of the cervix will feel softer and the opening will increase in size. You may also notice that the cervical opening has a slippery feeling which indicates that fertile fluid is being produced. These changes occur to facilitate the entry of sperm into the uterus and fallopian tubes. In its wisdom, the body will maintain this state only during times of potential conception. Having an open, penetrable cervix at all times leaves the uterus and other reproductive organs vulnerable to bacteria that could cause infection. Responding to hormonal changes, after ovulation, the cervix will again dip down and become tight and closed.

Cervical Fluid (CF)—Who Knew?

Though I had been treating infertility for years, it wasn't until studying for my American Board of Oriental Reproductive Medicine (ABORM) exam that I learned the intricate details of how CF changes in response to hormonal shifts throughout the menstrual cycle. Did you know there are four different kinds of CF, all produced by different cells in the cervix, signaled by changes in estrogen and progesterone? I didn't. Cervical fluid has a life of its own. Rather than being a passive player in conception, it's an active participant in achieving pregnancy. This type of body fluid changes several times during the menstrual cycle. It shifts consistency during your cycle to either block the cervix to outside invaders (be it sperm or bacteria) or nourish sperm and facilitate their movement towards a waiting egg.

Infertile CF is a barrier to protect the uterus. As ovulation approaches, the cervix starts to secrete fluids that are slick and slippery. This shift starts to occur (ideally) about six days prior to ovulation. Responding to increasing estrogen levels, the CF thins and becomes slippery. As the fluid first starts to change consistency, it allows only the strongest sperm to penetrate the uterine cavity. As estrogen levels increase, CF becomes slippery and stretchy. This fertile fluid forms a clear pathway for sperm to swim toward the egg. Finally, on the day of or just before ovulation, in addition to the stretchy "egg white" appearing mucus, the cervix secretes fluid that nourishes the sperm. This slippery, stretchy, wet mucus shows that you have reached the peak of your yin phase. As you shift to your yang phase, progesterone levels increase and the body's focus turns to warming the womb and supporting an embryo. This increased heat causes the CF to dry up. Post ovulation, CF becomes a dry, impenetrable barrier that protects the uterus and reproductive organs.

Becoming familiar with your CF patterns enables you to interpret your body's fertility signals during your cycle. However, just as there are factors that can throw off a BBT, there are also elements that can disrupt CF readings. For example: active yeast infections, the birth control pill, Clomid, NSAIDs, and anti-histamines will all inhibit or dry up CF. Serotonin Reuptake Inhibitors (SSRIs) like Prozac generally lessen CF. In some women, they actually promote CF.

You should have at least 3 days of wet, stretchy, clear or egg white CF. If not, there are some steps you can take to enhance it. Some practitioners advocate using guaifenesin (brand name, Mucinex) five days prior to ovulation to soften and alkalize CF. I have found that taking evening primrose oil, from day one through ovulation can dramatically improve the quality and quantity of CF. When treating my patients with Chinese formulas, I always include herbs that strengthen the yin and blood during the follicular phase, because they enhance CF and promote a high quality endometrium.

FAM Techniques: Summing It Up

When used correctly, the combination of BBT, CP and CF is highly effective in helping women pinpoint their fertile days. Once you know the week you are most fertile, be sure to have intercourse at least every other day that week up until the day after ovulation. You may certainly have intercourse before and after this time period, but it won't impact your chances of conception. Over a three month period, you can form an individual fertility profile to direct you towards heightened fertility. Furthermore, the effects of acupuncture, herbal formulas and a fertility friendly diet & lifestyle can impact the BBT in ways that are easy to recognize.

There are several BBT charts available for free online. You may also copy the blank BBT chart at the end of this chapter, though you will probably want to enlarge it. Be sure to track changes to your regular routine and other factors that can alter your chart so you can take them into consideration when evaluating the BBT at the end of the month. Notice that there is a space to track the results of LH surge predictor tests. I suggest to my patients that they combine FAM with LH surge predictors for more information on the exact time of ovulation. Also keep in mind that by itself, the BBT chart is not enough to *predict ovulation*. Some women are uncomfortable checking their CP, but you need to at least combine CF observations with the BBT for reliable fertility information.

There are several charts at the end of this chapter, labeled "Ovulation", "Anovulatory", "Endometriosis", "Pregnant" and one blank chart for you to copy and start the FAM. I included several examples from my practice along with Patient Notes to give you an idea of how different BBTs can look under different circumstances.

I hate doing this!

Most women embrace the FAM as a tool to learn about themselves and their unique fertility profile. This is especially true when they understand how tracking their temperatures can help them take control of their fertility. However, some women feel burdened by the task of taking their temperature each morning because it's a constant reminder that they are trying to get pregnant. Women whose BBT charts show no ovulation, or demonstrate other problems in the follicular and luteal phases, can become discouraged and depressed with the task. Of course, anxiety and stress are the opposite feelings of what we are trying to engender, which is becoming educated and empowered. So, other fertility monitoring tools may serve these women better.

Simply doing LH surge detection tests alone will yield some fertility information. These kits can be found at most drug stores and online. Ideally, the ovary will release an egg within 24-48 hours of the LH surge. I use the word 'ideally' because this test will simply tell you if the pituitary released enough LH to be detected in the urine, not how your ovaries reacted to it and if one released an egg. However, given that the ovaries respond appropriately, LH surge detectors are a relatively easy way to predict ovulation. In contrast to the FAM, this test is a "snapshot" in time, rather than a process oriented approach.

Another option for women who do not find the FAM feasible is the OV-Watch. The OV-Watch is worn nightly, starting on days 1-3 of your cycle and determines the most fertile days by measuring changes in the chemical composition of your perspiration. Just as hormonal shifts can be reflected in temperature changes, they can also change the salt makeup of perspiration. Through measuring changes in sweat, the OV-Watch claims to give a 5-6 day fertility window.

The OV-Watch is a good option for women who feel stressed out by BBT charting. They are available online through Amazon and other sites including: www.ovwatch.com. They cost around $100.00 and need the sensor replaced every month, which are sold separately. The OV-Watch yields a greater window of opportunity for conception than simply using LH surge kits alone. In fact, you can use the OV-Watch in addition to LH surge tests for even more information. The OV-Watch does not give information on the vitality of the follicular/yin phase or luteal/yang phase. Therefore, while it's a useful tool to predict ovulation, I still suggest the FAM to my patients first and propose the OV-Watch if the FAM is overwhelming, or for some reason impractical.

I did the FAM for two months and am really worried. Even though I took my temperature at the same time every morning, it bounced around between 96.1 and 97.2. There are no discernable "phases" or temperature shifts. The chart just looks like a sawtooth comb. What does this mean?

You may not be ovulating. Even if you are, your yin and yang phases are out of balance. So, the chances are low that you have built up the endometrium you need to nourish an embryo and sustain a pregnancy. If you were my patient, we would discuss your LH surge detector tests, any factors that could throw off the BBT and your CF. Then, I would discuss your options with you in terms of OM treatment and additional laboratory testing.

I've found Western laboratory and imaging tests to be an indispensable part of infertility diagnosis and treatment. For example, when Susan left my office after her initial visit, she had information on: fertility and nutrition, the FAM and a laboratory requisition to measure her LH, FSH, TSH, fT3, fT4, progesterone, estrogen and glucose. This was the first step to answering her question, "Am I healthy enough to get pregnant?"

Fertility is a marker of health. Some health issues do not come to light before trying to conceive, such as thyroid problems or polycystic ovary syndrome (PCOS). In the following chapter, we will talk about these and other issues that can make getting pregnant and having a healthy pregnancy more challenging.

Basal Body Temperature Chart—OVULATION

28 Year Old Woman With Polycystic Ovary Syndrome, After Five Months Of OM Treatment

Cycle Day	1	2	3	4	5	6	7	8	9	10	11	12	13	14	15	16	17	18	19	20	21	22	23	24	25	26	27	28	29	30	31	32	33	34	35	36	37	38	39	40	41	42	43	44	45
Date	1	2	3	4	5	6	7	8	9	10	11	12	13	14	15	16	17	18	19	20	21	22	23	24	25	26	27	28	29	30	1	2	3	4											
Time	8	7:30	7:30	8	7	6:30	6:30	6:30	5:30	6:30	6:30	6:30	6:30	6:30	6:30	8:30	6:30	6:30	6:30	6:30	8	6:30	6:30	6:30	6:30	6:30	8	6:30	6:30	7	6:30	6:30	6:30	6:30											

(Temperature grid, 99.1 – 96.9 °F, plotting Laura's basal body temperature across the cycle)

							X		X	X			X	X	X			X	X	X			X	X		X			X			X													
Intercourse							X		X	X			X	X	X			X	X	X			X	X		X			X			X													
Bleeding*	P	P	P	P	P																																								
CP*								L		L			L	L		H		H	H																										
CF*															E			E	S	S																									
LH Surge																		+																											

Notes:

Laura's BBT charts improved immediately after starting OM treatment. She was diligent about following her fertility enhancing diet, taking her herbal formulas and nutritional supplements, charting and having regular acupuncture sessions. Her work paid off. Notice these positive signs:

1. Her follicular phase temperatures don't vary by more than 0.3 degrees (when you adjust for the time she took her temperature)
2. She clearly has a low temperature followed by a dramatic spike indicating ovulation
3. Her CF and CP progression line up with her BBT, all three fertility indicators show that she ovulated and she had a positive LH surge
4. Her luteal phase temperatures remain elevated, they do not drop to pre-ovulation levels
5. She has a clear "thermal shift" between her follicular and luteal phases

*Bleeding (SP=Spotting, P=Period) *CF = Cervical Fluid (S=Stretchy, E=Egg White) *CP = Cervical Position: (L=Low, H=High)

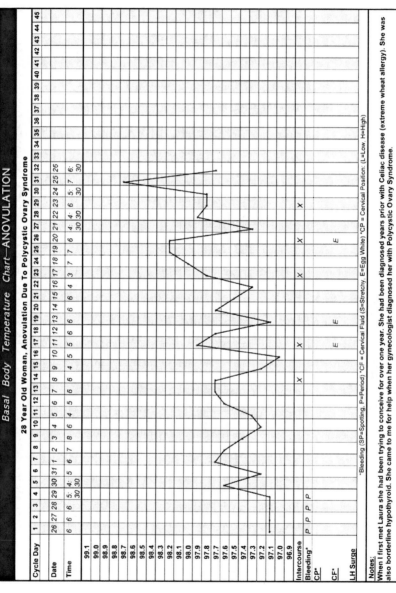

Basal Body Temperature Chart—ANOVULATION

28 Year Old Woman, Anovulation Due To Polycystic Ovary Syndrome

Notes:
When I first met Laura she had been trying to conceive for over one year. She had been diagnosed years prior with Celiac disease (extreme wheat allergy). She was also borderline hypothyroid. She came to me for help when her gynecologist diagnosed her with Polycystic Ovary Syndrome.

Laura had been charting her temperatures for almost one year. This was her most recent chart. She was very discouraged because it appears that she did not ovulate. Her temperatures are very erratic, even when you take the time she took her temperature into consideration.

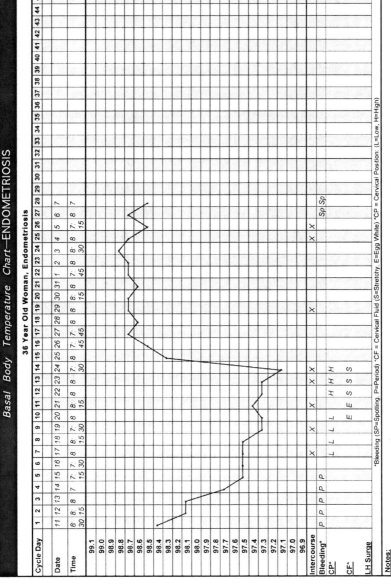

Basal Body Temperature Chart—ENDOMETRIOSIS

36 Year Old Woman, Endometriosis

Cycle Day	1	2	3	4	5	6	7	8	9	10	11	12	13	14	15	16	17	18	19	20	21	22	23	24	25	26	27	28	29	30	31	32	33	34	35	36	37	38	39	40	41	42	43	44	45
Date	11	12	13	14	15	16	17	18	19	20	21	22	23	24	25	26	27	28	29	30	31	1	2	3	4	5	6	7																	
Time	8: 30	8: 15	8	7	7: 15	7: 30	8	8: 15	7: 30	8: 15	8	8	8: 30	8	7: 45	7: 45	7: 45	8	8	8: 15	8: 45	7: 45	8	8: 30	8	7: 15	7: 8	7																	

Intercourse						X		X	X		X		X	X	X				X						X																				
Bleeding*	P	P	P	P	P																						Sp Sp																		
CP*								L	L	L	L	H	H	H																															
CF*										E	E	E	S	S	S																														
LH Surge																																													

*Bleeding (SP=Spotting, P=Period) *CF = Cervical Fluid (S=Stretchy, E=Egg White) *CP = Cervical Position: (L=Low, H=High)

Notes:
Paula came to me seeking help conceiving after one year of unprotected intercourse with her husband. Her BBT charts were very erratic, showing no discernable patterns of ovulation, follicular or luteal phases. She reported intense pain during the first two days of her period. Her laboratory tests showed low thyroid function. After a couple of months of OM treatment, her hypothyroid signs and symptoms diminished, BBT charts showed that she was ovulating. However, now the BBT chart indicated another problem. I suspect endometriosis when spotting starts prior to menstruation and the temperatures don't drop when menses starts. Paula wanted to combine OM with Intrauterine Insemination so I referred her to a reproductive endocrinologist. Unfortunately, he confirmed that Paula had endometriosis.

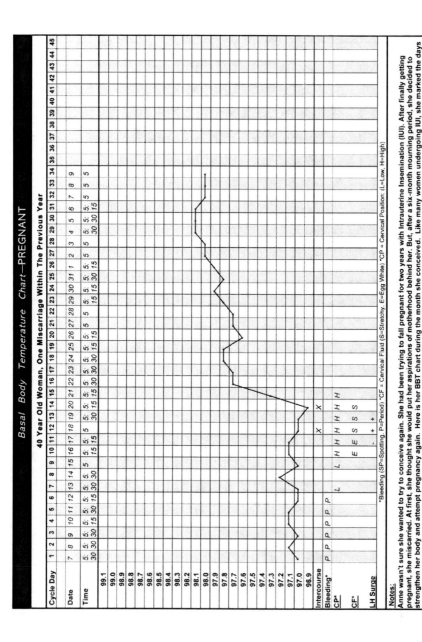

Basal Body Temperature Chart—PREGNANT

40 Year Old Woman, One Miscarriage Within The Previous Year

Notes:

Anne wasn't sure she wanted to try to conceive again. She had been trying to fall pregnant for two years with Intrauterine Insemination (IUI). After finally getting pregnant, she miscarried. At first, she thought she would put her aspirations of motherhood behind her. But, after a six-month mourning period, she decided to strengthen her body and attempt pregnancy again. Here is her BBT chart during the month she conceived. Like many women undergoing IUI, she marked the days she was inseminated in the "Intercourse" column.

As of this writing, Anne is eight months pregnant. She is scheduled to begin her "Pre-Birth Acupuncture Series" next month!

Basal Body Temperature Chart

Year

Month(s)

Cycle Day	1	2	3	4	5	6	7	8	9	10	11	12	13	14	15	16	17	18	19	20	21	22	23	24	25	26	27	28	29	30	31	32	33	34	35	36	37	38	39	40	41	42	43	44	45
Date																																													
Time																																													
99.1																																													
99.0																																													
98.9																																													
98.8																																													
98.7																																													
98.6																																													
98.5																																													
98.4																																													
98.3																																													
98.2																																													
98.1																																													
98.0																																													
97.9																																													
97.8																																													
97.7																																													
97.6																																													
97.5																																													
97.4																																													
97.3																																													
97.2																																													
97.1																																													
97.0																																													
96.9																																													
Intercourse																																													
Bleeding*																																													
CP*																																													
CF*																																													
LH Surge																																													

*Bleeding (SP=Spotting, P=Period) *CF = Cervical Fluid (S=Stretchy, E=Egg White) *CP = Cervical Position: (L=Low, H=High)

Notes: (List interfering factors such as: drugs, fevers, alcohol, insomnia and the dates)

Pregnancy and Fertility Challenges

FERTILITY IS A MEASURE of health and vitality. The ability to create and nourish new life, a new idea or a new direction in your life, with grace and fortitude, is directly related to the quality and quantity of your key resources: qi, blood, yin, yang and jing.

As we have discussed in previous chapters, there are several ways jing can be depleted; not the least of which is aging. Chemical exposure, stress, dietary choices and genetic tendencies also influence the way we utilize our resources. In this chapter, we explore some of the Western diagnosis often given to those struggling to conceive. We will discuss them from both Western and OM perspectives in terms of diagnosis, treatment options and potential impact on fertility and pregnancy. However, it is very important not to get wrapped up in a Western diagnosis. For example, just because you may have been diagnosed with endometriosis, this does not mean that you cannot conceive! Remember, you are an individual! You can make choices that impact your health on a daily basis. Your destiny is not set in stone, even if you have been told that you fall into one of the challenging categories discussed in this chapter.

Thyroid Imbalances

So far we've talked about the pituitary, ovaries, fallopian tubes, cervix and of course the UTERUS in regards to fertility, but what about that unsung hero, the thyroid gland? The thyroid gland sits in the front of your throat. It controls your whole body's metabolism—the metabolic activity of EVERY CELL! Because of this, thyroid disease affects every organ in the body, including reproductive organs.

Like the ovaries, the thyroid is controlled by the pituitary and the hypothalamus. When levels of thyroid hormone in the body drop, the pituitary sends a message to the thyroid via Thyroid Stimulating Hormone (TSH) to make more of the thyroid hormone, Thyroxine (T4). Like all of the hormonal pathways in the body, this is complicated!!! T4 has to be converted into a more bioactive hormone, Triiodothyronine (T3) to affect your cells and actually get anything accomplished. This conversion of T4 to T3 happens all over the body, but primarily in the liver. So, having optimal liver function is imperative for thyroid health.

The endocrine system is one big balancing act, so it stands to reason that it's possible to have too little of a hormone, and it is also to have too much. You can have too much estrogen, too much follicle stimulating hormone (FSH), not enough progesterone, etc. Thyroid hormones are no exception. Having too little thyroid hormone causes hypothyroidism, while having too much results in hyperthyroidism. Both hypo and hyperthyroidism can cause unpleasant symptoms, abnormal BBT fluctuations and imbalances in the key fertility hormones: FSH, LH, estrogen, progesterone, testosterone, cortisol, the list goes on and on… Additionally, hyperthyroidism and hypothyroidism can also be totally asymptomatic (present without showing symptoms) or subclinical (in early stages without discernable symptoms). As a result, fertility specialists often include thyroid tests in initial male and female fertility workups.

Hypothyroid Signs/Symptoms

- Weight gain and/or difficulty losing weight even with dieting and exercise
- Tendency to be cold
- High cholesterol
- Hair loss
- Depression
- Dry skin
- Memory & concentration difficulties
- Constipation
- Menstrual irregularities such as: unpredictable cycles, heavy bleeding and a history of miscarriage or stillbirths
- Basal body temperature readings may be low, so low that they don't register on the chart
- Temperature spikes may not demonstrate the relatively low valleys of the follicular phase and sustained peak of the luteal phase which indicates normal hormonal fluctuation and ovulation
- Rather than a bi-phasic chart showing a yin phase followed by a yang phase, one may see a sawtooth pattern where it becomes impossible to determine when and if ovulation occurred

Hyperthyroid Signs/Symptoms

- Unexplained weight loss
- Anxiety
- Insomnia
- Restlessness
- Shaking
- Thirst
- Exopthalmos (an eye condition resulting in bulging and irritation)

- Shortness of breath
- Basal body temperatures measurements may be chronically elevated or sawtooth
- Temperature shifts showing ovulation may also be absent

While hypothyroidism and hyperthyroidism are opposite sides of the spectrum, both of these conditions may present symptoms of fatigue and muscle pain or weakness.

How does this impact my fertility?

Now for the part you have been waiting for. Yes, this is all very interesting information, but how is taking care of your thyroid going to help you GET (AND STAY) PREGNANT!?

Both hyper and hypothyroidism can result in anovulation (the absence of ovulation). Of course if you are not ovulating, you won't be getting pregnant. Plus, if you have thyroid disease and do get pregnant, the baby could suffer, becoming either hypo or hyperthyroid itself. Hypothyroidism in early pregnancy can negatively affect the developing baby's brain and nervous system. Children born to mothers with hypothyroidism during pregnancy can struggle in school and suffer from lower IQs. On the other hand, hyperthyroidism can be toxic to the baby. If the mother's thyroid condition is caused by an autoimmune problem, the mother could be hyperthyroid while the baby is hypothyroid!

Yin and Yang Disharmony, an Ancient Name for Hyper and Hypothyroidism
Chinese researchers examined 109 patients with either hyperthyroid or hypothyroid conditions and diagnosed them according to Chinese medicine principals. Each participant had TSH, T3 and T4 blood laboratory tests. Interestingly, scientists found that the diagnosis of yin deficiency corresponded to hyperthyroidism (low TSH, high T3 and T4) while hypothyroid (high TSH and low T3 and T4) subjects displayed a yang deficient pattern.

I have a lot of hypothyroid symptoms. What should I do?

Thyroid disease can easily go undiagnosed and have serious effects on fertility and a developing baby. If you suspect that you have a thyroid problem, either because of your BBT or you have more than 3 symptoms of thyroid disturbance, contact your primary health care provider and request a thyroid workup. An initial screening test is an inexpensive, simple blood test that measures the amount of TSH in your body. Depending on your symptoms, your physician may also order tests that directly measure levels of thyroid hormones and thyroid antibodies. Interpreting these tests is both art and science. Sometimes tests will be borderline rather than obviously conclusive and the physician must make a clinical evaluation based on symptoms and desired fertility outcome.

Of course, you want to minimize your exposure to substances that can have a harmful effect on thyroid function, such as chemical pollutants that mimic or alter hormone function, and iodine levels in the body. If you have an overactive thyroid, follow a diet geared towards minimizing inflammation. If you tend towards hypothyroidism, supplementing your diet with sea vegetables such as kelp and hijiki with provide you with good quality iodine.

We will discuss this topic further in the Fertility Friendly Diet & Lifestyle chapter. Additionally, several Western herbs, acupuncture, Chinese herbal formulas, nutritional supplements and thyroid hormones may be used to normalize your thyroid and improve fertility. A holistic physician well versed in fertility should be able to guide you in choosing the best treatment for you.

Endometriosis

You may have heard of endometriosis. Perhaps a girlfriend or sister with painful periods told you she was diagnosed with it. This would not be surprising as endometriosis affects millions of women of childbearing age. What's more, over half of these women experience fertility difficulties. Some women with endometriosis experience persistent, severe menstrual cramping, spotting throughout the month - especially a few days before their period. They may also suffer from painful intercourse, urination and defecation. One of my most experienced Chinese gynecology teachers told me that women who cramp after their periods also have endometriosis. On the other hand, many women diagnosed with this disease report no symptoms other than infertility. No one really knows the cause of endometriosis, though it is widely speculated that a faulty immune system, genetics, high fat diets, long term lack of exercise, hormone imbalances, environmental toxins and stress are all contributing factors.

What IS endometriosis?

In short, endometriosis is endometrial tissue (the lining of the uterus in which an embryo can implant) outside of the uterus. Theoretically, endometrial lesions can be anywhere in the body but are most commonly found in the abdominal cavity. This tissue can implant on ovaries, fallopian tubes, the bladder and bowels. When endometriosis adheres to the ovaries, (endometriomas) it can be particularly deleterious to fertility. Even though the endometrial cells are outside of the uterus, they still respond to estrogen and progesterone. This causes swelling and bleeding in the abdominal cavity, which can result in great pain, scarring and adhesions that can distort the reproductive organs...in some women. Other women experience absolutely no symptoms.

The Puzzle of Endometriosis

The severity of endometriosis is graded as mild, moderate or severe. Intuitively, it makes sense that women with severe disease show scarring and distortion of the fallopian tubes, ovaries or uterus, experience pain and infertility. However, some women with very mild endometriosis, meaning there is very little endometrial tissue outside of the uterus, can have extreme pain and infertility, while other women with severe disease have no pelvic pain or trouble falling pregnant. Why? No one really knows.

In fact, Western researchers are not even sure what causes endometriosis or exactly how it interferes with fertility. "Retrograde menstruation", proposed in 1927, was the first theory to explain endometriosis. Uterine contractions during menstruation should cause endometrial tissue to flow out the cervix and through the vagina. Retrograde menstruation is the term for menstrual blood that backflows up through the fallopian tubes and into the abdomen. Ideally, the body should absorb this tissue. If it does not, abdominal blood stasis can result, causing endometriosis.

Another theory holds that the immune system plays a pivotal role in the development and progression of endometriosis. On one hand, the immune system should keep endometrial tissue from implanting outside the uterus. On the other hand, once endometriosis develops, the immune system can make antibodies to this tissue, causing inflammation and hormonal imbalances, which can hinder egg implantation, cause recurrent miscarriages and even kill sperm!

There is also a strong genetic component to endometriosis. If your mother or sisters have it, you are at greater risk for developing it. Perhaps you were born with endometrial tissue outside of your uterus, which lay dormant until you hit puberty. This predisposition combined with high amounts of stress, exposure to hormonally active environmental toxins (xenoestrogens) that can increase your estrogen levels, a high body mass index (BMI) and suboptimal liver function could tip the balance and cause you to develop this disease. (To find out more about xenoestrogens, and how to determine your BMI, see the Fertility Friendly Diet & Lifestyle chapter.)

Ironically, there is evidence that endometriosis both **results from and causes** immune and endocrine system problems which make it more difficult to conceive and hold a pregnancy. Women with endometriosis can have a shorter, less functional luteal phase due to faulty progesterone secretion and metabolism, which can cause early miscarriage and infertility. Another irony is that stress can cause elevations in the hormones cortisol and prolactin, which research shows are higher in women with severe endometriosis. High levels of these hormones can upset your hormonal balance, causing more stress, increased hormonal chaos, and so on.

This sounds really, really complicated and I'm concerned that I may have endometriosis. WHERE should I start?

First, evaluate your chances of having endometriosis. How many of the signs and symptoms of endometriosis do you have?

Endometriosis Signs/Symptoms & Risk Factors

- Painful periods
- Intense cramping may start 1-2 days prior to menstruation and can be so severe that it causes vomiting, diarrhea and fainting
- Pain at the end of, or just AFTER menses
- Irregular anovulatory cycles
- Irregular menstrual spotting
- Painful intercourse
- History of sexual abuse
- High levels of stress
- High serum levels of prolactin, cortisol and/or the presence of autoantibodies
- Prior use of intra-uterine devices (IUDs)
- Close female relative with endometriosis
- Infertility
- BBT graph abnormalities such as: the temperature does not drop significantly at the beginning of the period, or it may drop, but then rises again during menstrual bleeding. Another abnormal BBT pattern associated with endometriosis is that after ovulation the temperature takes several days to rise, or it rises but then falls again in a few days during the ovulation phase.

Evaluate Your Options

I would be remiss to advise women with pelvic pain to forgo a gynecological exam. Women with endometriosis often experience lower abdominal and reproductive organ tenderness with a pelvic exam. Adhesions, enlarged ovaries, and an immobile or "tipped" uterus may be detectable. While a clinician may suspect endometriosis from a patient's history and exam, a laparoscopy is the only definitive way to make this diagnosis.

What is a laparoscopy?

Laparoscopic treatment is the standard Western test procedure for women with suspected endometriosis who wish to conceive. While the patient is under general anesthesia, her abdomen is filled with gas and a scope is inserted through a small cut in or around her navel. Through this scope, the physician examines the reproductive organs. Typically, a second incision is made beneath the pubic line so the surgeon can move the organs for better viewing. If endometriosis or adhesions are found, they can be removed during this procedure. Laparoscopy is touted to be both diagnostic and when ablation of endometriosis is added, therapeutic. Indeed, fertility rates in women whose reproductive organs have been distorted by endometriosis can improve for the next several months or years after laparoscopy. Women under 35 are most likely to experience this benefit. As always, results vary with every individual. Sometimes endometriosis is difficult to see, it may be a whitish or pink color and therefore the surgeon can miss it. Alternately, it may have caused cysts on the ovaries, leaving the surgeon with the difficult decision of whether or not to remove the endometriomas and potentially damage the ovary resulting in less available follicles. In women with mild endometriosis, reports conflict in terms of the efficacy of performing laparoscopy with ablation. Some experts say it improves pregnancy rates, while others assert that not only is it unhelpful, it may even reduce fertility!

What other Western therapies are available?

Western medicine offers treatment in the form of narcotics or non-steroidal anti-inflammatories (NSAIDs) such as naproxen or ibuprophen. There is some evidence that taking anti-inflammatories mid-cycle can prevent ovulation, so for the management of infertility related endometriosis these drugs are prescribed just prior to and during menstruation. Another protocol consists of hormone therapy to "starve" the endometriosis of nutrients, hopefully resulting in repression of the disease. Because hormonal regimens are geared towards halting endometrial growth, they are not indicated for women who are trying to conceive. Additionally, they can cause a number of very unpleasant side effects such as hot flashes, reduced libido, amenorrhea, acne, weight gain, nausea, headaches, muscle cramps and facial hair. Sometimes women with documented endometriosis will be placed on hormonal therapy as part of an IVF protocol (see the Assisted Reproductive Techniques chapter) in the hope that this additional hormonal regulation will increase the chances of pregnancy.

Given the shortfalls of Western medical treatment options for endometriosis, it's not surprising that more and more women are turning towards OM for pain reduction and fertility enhancement.

What can OM offer me for the treatment of endometriosis?

Women with endometriosis often have a difficult time shifting from yang to yin and yin to yang during the phases of their menstrual cycle. Premenstrual spotting and irregular BBT charts are signs of this imbalance. OM therapy for endometriosis is therefore applied to ease these transitions by both correcting the underlying causes of disharmony (such as deficient qi, blood, yang or jing) and by moving qi and blood. Typically, practitioners use a combination of acupuncture, herbal formulas and dietary therapy to accomplish these goals. The main focus of OM treatment is to enhance circulation and reduce inflammation to restore the pelvic and reproductive organs to normal functioning. One key strengths of OM is that many factors are taken into account to establish a cohesive picture, rather than trying to identify ONE specific CAUSE of a disease and "fixing" that single cause. The pieces to the endometriosis puzzle fit together best when we look at what grade and type of endometriosis is present and how the body responds to it. Only by performing an individual diagnosis and treatment plan can a practitioner comprise a dynamic treatment strategy to treat this condition and enhance fertility.

Endometriosis: Pieces of the Puzzle
Researchers in Japan measured levels of Immunoglobulin M antibodies and estrogen in women with endometriosis. They then divided these women into two groups, one group received hormone therapy and the other was treated with a traditional OM formula. Interestingly, while the hormonal therapy group's estrogen levels dropped, their antibody levels remained the same. The OM group's estrogen levels remained the same but their antibodies dropped and their symptoms disappeared for over six months.

Where do the needles go?

Many women with endometriosis experience severe pelvic pain. They resist trying acupuncture for fear that the needles will go right where it already hurts. Who could blame them? But, not to worry. While there are several points on the abdomen used for promoting fertility such as Zi Gong (translated as "baby palace") there are also plenty of points to choose from in other areas of the body. In my practice I never place a needle into a spasming muscle group. That could cause more pain! When I see women in acute menstrual pain, I use acupuncture points with pain relieving properties on the hands, feet and lower legs. There are also different types of acupuncture to choose from. For example, Japanese style acupuncture is known for its gentle needle techniques. Often patients don't even feel the needles at all! Other options for pain relief include using a hot pack or placing moxabustion on the abdomen during treatment. It is very important to honor the fact that endometriosis can be very painful and not insist on sticking a needle where it hurts!

Japanese Acupuncture & Endometriosis
Researchers at Harvard medical school conducted a small study looking at the effect of Japanese style acupuncture on endometriosis induced chronic pelvic pain in young women. The group who received Japanese acupuncture demonstrated a significant pain reduction at the end of the study.

How do herbs help women with endometriosis?

Herbal treatment of women with endometriosis who are trying to get pregnant is not significantly different than the herbal treatment of anyone trying to get pregnant. Different formulas that enhance each phase of the cycle are given during those phases. During the period, herbal formulas are given to reduce pain and increase blood circulation in order to promote a smooth transition from yang to yin. After menses stops, blood and yin tonifying herbs are taken to support hormonal balance and proper uterine lining formation. Key to the herbal treatment of endometriosis is herbal administration mid-cycle to facilitate ovulation and move qi to enable yin to transform to yang. Then, formulas that support the yang and gently move blood are prescribed during the luteal phase to enhance the metabolic activity of the womb and increase the likelihood of embryonic implantation. If there is no embryo, then yang should smoothly transform back to yin when the period comes. Given proper treatment during the beginning of the cycle, yang should shift smoothly to yin on its own. If there is a pregnancy, the herbs used in the yang part of the cycle should assist the body in retaining the pregnancy. Particular to endometriosis treatment is focusing on moving blood and relieving pain during menses.

Is there any research to support the use of herbs in treating endometriosis?

Yes, there is. While it is not possible to fully research the energetic phenomenon of assisting 'yin and yang transformation', we can study the chemical components of individual herbs and the actions of OM formulas. Several herbal medicinals traditionally known to 'move qi and blood' have been the subject of Western research in endometriosis and painful periods (dysmenorrhea). Many of these herbs tested in both humans and animals demonstrate anti-inflammatory, muscle relaxant and anti-oxidant effects. For example, turmeric and white peony root have a long history of use in OM for dysmenorrhea. Current research shows these herbs possess antioxidant, anti-inflammatory and pain reducing properties.

In traditional Chinese herbalism, single herbs are rarely used. Rather, they are combined together in ways that augment their properties to induce synergistic effects. In a typical formula for endometriosis, not just one, but several herbs with anti-inflammatory, anti-oxidant and muscle relaxant effects are used for treatment.

Women with endometriosis who want to get pregnant don't have to stick with just Eastern or just Western treatments. Many women combine Western and OM treatments.

Integrated Medicine: East PLUS West, Increases Fertility and Reduces Pain for Women with Endometriosis

To study various treatments for advanced endometriosis, researchers in China divided 152 infertile women with ovarian endometrial cysts into three groups: one group took Chinese herbal medicine, one group received Danazol (hormone treatment) while the last group took Chinese herbs after having a laparoscopy. Women in the last group had the greatest reduction in endometriosis symptoms AND the highest pregnancy rate.

Polycystic Ovary Syndrome (PCOS)

PCOS is a leading cause of infertility. It's the most common endocrine disorder afflicting women. The good news is that many women with PCOS conceive and deliver healthy babies.

One doctor said I have PCOS, but another one said I didn't. I am so confused. I don't really even understand what PCOS is.

Each month during the follicular phase, under the guidance of FSH and the influence of estrogen, several follicles containing immature eggs start to develop. Typically, only the strongest follicle reaches maturity and releases its egg while the others wither. Not so in a woman with PCOS. Due to a complex interplay of faulty blood sugar metabolism and hormonal dysregulation the ovarian follicles are arrested in their development. Thus, in women with PCOS, ovulation is irregular, unpredictable or non-existent. On ultrasound the ovarian cysts (which really aren't cysts, but partially developed follicles) look like a string of pearls.

We know that PCOS is very common, affecting between 6-10% of premenopausal women. In fact, it is the most prevalent cause of anovulatory (no ovulation) infertility in the developing world. However, it is difficult to say exactly how widespread PCOS is because this syndrome is so complex. Only recently have Western experts reached a consensus as to the defining signs and symptoms of PCOS. In a meeting between the European Society of Human Reproduction and Embryology (ESHRE) and the American Society for Reproductive Medicine (ASRM) in 2004, the definition of PCOS was set as being: **two out of three key symptoms: infrequent or absent menstrual periods, specific hormonal imbalances and polycystic ovaries.**

Infrequent or Absent Menstrual Periods

Most women with PCOS don't completely stop menstruating. They tend to have long cycles with 6-8 menstrual periods per year. This is due to infrequent ovulation, which of course decreases the likelihood of conception.

Hormonal Imbalances

Women with PCOS have a disruption in the yin and yang phases of their cycle. They don't have a full and complete yin phase to support a healthy yang phase. In other words, women with PCOS are locked into the follicular phase. Biochemically this can manifest as too little estrogen, too much testosterone, high LH, low sex hormone binding globulin (SHBG) as well as many other endocrine abnormalities. These hormone irregularities can cause problems beyond infertility. Because of their negative affect on the quality of developing eggs, they can increase the chances of miscarriage, whether conception occurred naturally or through artificial reproductive techniques (ART).

There are many theories as to why some women develop these hormonal imbalances. The tendency could be inherited. Indeed, women with close female relatives with PCOS are at higher risk for developing the disorder. Current thinking asserts that women who are prone to developing PCOS are also more likely to have blood sugar abnormalities. It is a vicious cycle where one problem gives rise to and exacerbates the other. Overweight women, as defined by a BMI greater than 30, are more likely to have faulty blood sugar metabolism, which can affect their reproductive hormones (you can calculate your BMI by using the table in the Diet and Lifestyle chapter).

Therefore, achieving a BMI between 19 and 24 by having a diet that focuses on maintaining stable blood sugar levels is one key to boosting fertility in these women. Briefly, the hormone that controls cellular uptake of glucose is insulin. When the body is flooded with glucose, especially after a meal or snack high in simple carbohydrates, insulin rises. Problems occur when women get locked into a state of high insulin (hyperinsulinemia). This state that can create hormonal problems in the ovaries resulting in abnormal egg development and infertility.

The String of Pearls

The last definitive criteria of PCOS is polycystic ovaries. An ultrasound will show 12 or more small cysts (remember these really aren't cysts in the true sense, they are immature follicles containing eggs) which look like a string of pearls sitting on top of the ovaries.

So, if my doctor tells me that I have polycystic ovaries, then I have PCOS, right?

No. You need two out of three diagnostic criteria to qualify for this disorder. That means that some women have PCOS without actually having polycystic ovaries. Plus, up to 1/3 of all women have polycystic ovaries. These women also have normal hormone levels, normal menstruation patterns and no fertility issues. So, PCOS **is not** synonymous with polycystic ovaries.

There are several reasons it took so many years for Western specialists to define PCOS. This complex syndrome can manifest in many different ways. Five women with PCOS may have completely different blood test results, family histories and ovarian ultrasounds.

PCOS Signs/Symptoms & Risk Factors

- Polycystic ovaries
- Infrequent, absent or irregular menstrual periods
- High testosterone levels
- Low SHBG
- Twice the blood level of LH as compared with FSH when measured in the first few days of the menstrual cycle
- Insulin resistance
- BMI >25
- Excessive facial hair (hirsutism)
- Acne
- Male pattern hair loss
- Spots of dark skin, especially on the face (acanthosis nigricans)
- Infertility
- Recurrent miscarriage

How did I get it?

That's a simple question with a complicated answer. There are several theories attempting to explain the onset and progression of PCOS. Both OM and Western medical perspectives center on the interplay of nature and nurture in PCOS development.

Nature (Genetics/Fetal Life/Pre-heaven Essence)

According to Western scientists, you may have inherited a predisposition to developing PCOS. Animal studies show that female babies exposed in utero to the type of hormonal imbalances common in PCOS are more likely to manifest PCOS in adolescence and adulthood. This exposure could have come from faulty gene expression. A gene involved with insulin metabolism has been linked to infertility from PCOS. We know that pregnant women with faulty blood sugar metabolism, whether it's from diet and lifestyle factors, hormonal imbalances or liver and pancreas dysfunction are more likely to pass PCOS to their daughters. Additionally, females born to obese mothers or who had a high birth weight or a long gestation (were overdue) are at a higher risk for developing PCOS. Lastly, it is clear that your chances of developing PCOS are higher if your mother or sisters have it.

Now let's look at the development of PCOS from an OM viewpoint. As with any fertility challenge, the root is in the Kidneys. Remember from Chapter 1 that the Kidneys govern our pre-heaven essence, our genetics. As such, they are the foundation of all of our yin and yang. They guide us through the rhythm of yin and yang transformation during the menstrual cycle. In PCOS, a deficiency of jing, Kidney yin or Kidney yang can cause this normal rhythm to become disrupted, resulting in incomplete egg maturation, absence of ovulation, irregular cycles and infertility.

Nurture (Lifestyle Choices/Post-heaven Essence)

While you can't control your genes, how long you were in the womb, if your mother had PCOS or what she ate while she was pregnant, you CAN control *your* lifestyle. As with most causes of infertility, (except actual birth defects) diet and lifestyle choices can determine the degree to which your inherited potential traits express themselves. This is where the Spleen, as the foundation of our post-heaven essence, comes into play. In general, a Spleen friendly diet focuses on a low glycemic index (meals that won't spike your blood sugar, discussed in the Diet and Lifestyle chapter) of dishes which include few cold or raw foods. Exercise also helps the Spleen perform better, as it moves qi, reduces stress and regulates the neuroendocrine system. There is growing evidence that demonstrates the negative impact of stress on PCOS (and the mediating effects that acupuncture and exercise can produce). Additionally, if the Spleen is not functioning optimally, blood sugar imbalances and faulty body fluid production are more likely to occur. As we discussed, blood sugar irregularities can cause hormonal fluctuations (an unhealthy Spleen disrupting Kidney function) and cause unhealthy variations in body fluids such as: thick cervical mucus at ovulation, dense fallopian tube secretions and ovarian cysts.

The first line therapy in both Western and OM is diet and lifestyle improvement. In women with a BMI over 25, losing just 5-10 lbs can jump-start ovulation and boost fertility.

Laura's Story

Laura, a slightly overweight, 28 year old woman, had her first visit with me after trying to fall pregnant for six years. She had been charting her temperature for about one year, and upon receiving a PCOS diagnosis from her gynecologist, tried clomiphene citrate (trade name Clomid). *She responded to Clomid, and ovulated, but didn't get pregnant. Without Clomid, her BBT charts, LH to FSH ratio, negative midcycle LH surge detector tests and irregular menses all indicated that she was not ovulating. You can see Laura's "Anovulatory" chart at the end of the previous chapter.*

Interestingly, Laura's mother, Claire, starting receiving treatment from me during the same time period for migraines and nausea. I was struck by how similar Laura and Claire looked. Laura told me that it took her mother years of trying before she conceived Laura. In fact, it wasn't until Claire took Clomid that she fell pregnant with her only child, Laura.

Since Laura had been trying to conceive for several years, she already had done quite a bit of research on PCOS and fertility. She knew that her diet was critical. Several years prior she had been diagnosed with Celiac disease (severe gluten intolerance). Even though she did her best to avoid wheat products, she still had intense abdominal pain, gas, bloating, constipation and overall poor digestion. During our first visit we talked about the importance of avoiding sugar in addition to wheat. It wasn't until several weeks later that I learned that she had a bakery. She was making wheat free treats—WITH SUGAR!

I laughed out loud when she told me this. My usual professional demeanor vanished, as I was so surprised. At first she was hurt and thought I was laughing AT her. I was not. I was laughing at the absurdity of the situation. I have an extensive medical history intake, and spend a lot of time with patients during the first and subsequent visits in an effort to root out all of the contributing factors to their disease process. I laughed because it took quite a while to uncover this fact and it was SO pivotal!

By the end of the visit we were both laughing. She stopped eating sugar; in fact she gave up her bakery business. She worked very hard implementing substantial changes in her diet and lifestyle, taking herbal formulas and nutritional supplements, receiving acupuncture treatments and doing the FAM. She followed the FAM to the letter. Not only did she take her temperature every morning, she learned how taking her temperature at different times affected her chart, she learned to interpret her CF and CP. In short, she discovered how to read the fertility signals her body was giving her. Within five months of treatment she had lost weight and was ovulating every month on a consistent basis (see Laura's "Ovulation" chart in the previous chapter).

What caused Laura's PCOS? Was it nature or nurture? Did she inherit a gene that affected her insulin metabolism? Is this how she developed in a hyperinsulinemic, testosterone rich environment? Or did she simply eat too much wheat and sugar? In Laura's case, I think it was a combination of all of these factors, pre and post-heaven influences. But, in a way, it really doesn't matter how she got PCOS. What matters is that she took control of her health by learning about her body and changing what she could. Now she is ovulating on a regular basis and if she conceives a girl, her daughter will likely have a smaller chance of developing PCOS.

But, I'm thin.

I have had so many women come to me claiming to have PCOS, even through their MD assured them it was not possible. They were "too skinny to have PCOS". Unfortunately, there is a widely held notion that women with PCOS are all overweight.

Women can be underweight (BMI<18) and have PCOS. In these cases, the underlying cause may be irregular activity by the pituitary, adrenal gland, the ovaries, or it could STILL be insulin resistance. It is important to remember that being too thin doesn't help fertility, either. Treatment options have to be carefully considered for thin women with insulin resistance, since losing weight isn't going to enhance their fertility.

If my MD thinks I have PCOS, what help can she offer me?

In terms of drug interventions you may be able to select from a few different options. While the drugs differ, the intent is the same: to push ovulation. For more details about the different hormone therapies used to boost fertility, see the Assisted Reproductive Techniques (ART) chapter.

Clomid is often prescribed to women with PCOS to enhance follicular growth and ovulation. By interfering with the communication between the ovaries, pituitary and hypothalamus, Clomid floods the body with FSH. Ideally, this leads to the development of a couple of follicles and ovulation, and of course pregnancy. Indeed, research shows Clomid can increase pregnancy rates in women afflicted with PCOS. Typically, Clomid therapy is more successful in women with a BMI lower than 30.

While Clomid can cause ovulation in women with PCOS, it does have a few shortcomings. There is an 11% increased chance of multiple pregnancies and a 23.6% miscarriage rate. Clomid can inhibit cervical fluid secretion and diminish endometrial lining. So, while it may help you ovulate, the sperm may not reach the oocyte. Even if conception occurs, the embryo may not be able to implant.

Another drawback is Clomid's effect on LH production. Too much LH too early in the cycle can decrease the chances of conception and if conception does occur, increases the risk of miscarriage. In some women, Clomid can trigger premature LH secretion. Women with PCOS are especially susceptible to this problem because they may already tend towards an abnormally high follicular phase LH level. When LH surges too early in the cycle, the yin is not fully allowed to develop before yang asserts itself, causing a yin and yang imbalance.

If Clomid does not yield the desired result, another class of hormones, gonadotropins (several types and brands available), may be prescribed. While Clomid influences the hypothalamus, gonadotropins work directly on the ovaries to encourage egg maturation. These are the most common drugs used in IVF cycles. They are considerably stronger than Clomid and therefore yield greater chances of both success and dangerous side effects.

These hormonal treatments sound strong. What can I expect in terms of side effects?

There are several common, though not dangerous, symptoms associated with these drugs such as night sweats, abdominal pain, headaches, nausea, vomiting and hot flashes.

However, there can be some serious side effects. Women with PCOS can be very sensitive to hormonal manipulation because they already produce several developing follicles. Their ovaries can overreact to the stimulation. Therefore, women with PCOS have a higher than average risk of developing a serious complication called ovarian hyperstimulation syndrome (OHSS). In OHSS, too many follicles are activated, which can result in fluid accumulation in the abdomen and in severe cases, the pericardium and lungs. Common symptoms of OHSS include nausea, vomiting, difficulty breathing and abdominal distention. This situation can be fatal and hospitalization to drain the excess fluid may be required. Other, more severe conditions associated with gonadotropin use are pregnancies that take place outside of the uterus (ectopic pregnancies) and ovarian twisting (adnexal torsion). Both of these complications may require surgery.

Since many women's PCOS is rooted in insulin problems, what if I just skip all the hormones and take a pill to help stabilize my blood sugar? Then I'll be more fertile, right?

In a word, no. The drug metformin is commonly prescribed to PCOS patients to regulate blood sugar metabolism. It works by both decreasing insulin levels and making cells more sensitive to insulin. Through regulating your body's blood sugar, metformin can help restore normal hormone levels and regulate menstruation.

Ok, that sounds good. I want a metformin prescription!

Yes, normal hormone levels and regular menses are important, but we're also interested in fertility! The first studies examining the relationship between metformin and PCOS suggested that metformin could significantly improve fertility. Unfortunately, larger more controlled studies have failed to show this. Clomid proved to be far more effective in promoting ovulation in PCOS patients. According to a study sponsored by the National Institutes of Health, adding metformin to Clomid yielded very little benefit. Additionally, another study published in the *Journal of Obstetrics and Gynecology* showed that metformin was no better than a placebo in both markedly overweight women with a BMI greater than 32, and in women with a BMI under 32. It was also found that women in the thinner group responded better to Clomid and had a higher number of pregnancies and live births.

Is there any other effective Western treatment that will help me ovulate on my own where I don't have to take hormones or change my lifestyle?

Yes. There is an alternative to drug treatment and lifestyle changes. It won't cause multiple pregnancies or give you OHSS. It is surgery. Ovarian diathermy is a procedure where small sections of ovaries are cauterized by electricity or laser. This injures the ovary and seems to "push the reset button" resulting in a higher sensitivity to FSH, lower testosterone levels and increased pregnancy rates. Scientists are unsure of exactly why this works. Some speculate that it reduces the effect of the sympathetic nervous system on ovarian function (just like acupuncture!). On the downside, this procedure destroys parts of the ovary and may lead to ovarian failure.

O.K., it seems that Western medicine has some options for me. How can OM help me?

It is important to keep in mind that PCOS is a Western diagnosis that can manifest in many different ways. In OM, receiving an individualized diagnosis is paramount to successful treatment. Women with PCOS are best served when practitioners take into account lab work, imaging reports and OM diagnosis when formulating a treatment protocol. In this next section we will look at OM's long history of ovulation induction and some of the current research on acupuncture, physical exercise, herbal formulas and PCOS.

Women with PCOS get stuck in the yin phase of the cycle, unable to make the shift into the yang phase through ovulation. This commonly manifests as yin deficiency (where there isn't enough yin to give rise to the yang phase) or dampness (an accumulation of turbid yin and sticky body fluids which blocks ovulation and yang transformation). This inability for yin to switch to yang mid-cycle has been the subject of Chinese scholars throughout the history of OM. A great deal has been written about it since gynecology became a specialty in the 8th century C.E. At that time in China, it was believed that part of every woman's destiny was to give birth and raise children. While pigeonholing all women in this role sounds chauvinistic today, the medical scholars of the time held a great regard for women. Therefore, they were at the forefront of fertility enhancement. Promoting ovulation, conception and preventing miscarriage was the work of OM gynecologists with reverence towards women.

Acupuncture Treatment for PCOS

Modern Chinese medical writings on ovulation induction using acupuncture and moxabustion began in the 1960s. At this time, acupuncture was used in hospitals in rural areas of China with a success rate between 30-50%. The points used were located on the Spleen, Kidney, and Liver meridians to address both prenatal and postnatal causes of anovulation. Since that time, a great deal of research has been done on the influence of acupuncture on PCOS.

Ways in Which Acupuncture Treatment Can Help PCOS
- Normalizing hormone levels
- Mediating the sympathetic nervous system
- Reducing acne and histurism
- Promoting ovulation and regular menstruation
- Improving pregnancy rates
- Encouraging weight loss by regulating insulin related gene expression
- Enhancing insulin sensitivity and decreasing glucose and insulin levels
- Increasing ovarian blood flow while decreasing the number of ovarian cysts

Several studies show that acupuncture significantly increases endorphin levels and can have a regulatory effect on FSH, LH and androgen (testosterone and other male hormones) levels. One of the proposed mechanisms of acupuncture's action on hormone levels is that it influences the hypothalamic-pituitary-adrenal (APA) axis. More simply stated, acupuncture can change the way the organs in your endocrine system work together, resulting in positive changes in hormone levels.

The endocrine system is affected by a myriad of factors. One of those factors is the state of the nervous system, especially the delicate balance between the sympathetic and parasympathetic parts of the nervous system. You have probably heard of these systems before. They are often referred to as the "fight or flight" and "rest and digest" aspects of the nervous system. The sympathetic nervous system kicks into gear when you feel stressed, for example, during morning traffic when you're late to work. The parasympathetic nervous system, in contrast, is dominant when you feel relaxed, for instance, after eating dinner on a calm evening. A healthy libido requires a complex interaction of both parts of the nervous system.

The sympathetic nervous system affects the uterus and ovaries in a restrictive way. The activation of the "fight or flight" response directs blood flow away from reproductive organs and out to the extremities, so you can fight or run away! It also triggers the release of the stress hormone cortisol and triggers the body to pour glucose into the blood. It was very important in our evolution to develop this stress response. In our modern society, this life-or-death response isn't usually activated by a stalking tiger, but by deadlines and similar stresses. These responses happen not once a week or once a month, but daily.

International Research on PCOS

Many current, important studies on acupuncture and reproductive medicine originate in Sweden. One such study examined the relationship between PCOS and the sympathetic nervous system. Scientists found that acupuncture can affect PCOS by regulating the sympathetic nervous, endocrine and neuroendocrine systems. Thus, acupuncture can redirect blood to the uterus and ovaries!

We have established that an overactive sympathetic nervous system contributes to the onset and exacerbation of PCOS. What can shift this pattern? Acupuncture, of course, but what about exercise or diet? How do these interventions compare to acupuncture treatment? To answer these questions, researchers studied the effects of diet, exercise and acupuncture on PCOS. They found that exercise, dietary changes and consistent acupuncture treatments improve the symptoms of PCOS including: testosterone and estrogen levels, menstrual frequency, acne, histruism, and pregnancy rates. Commenting on the significance of their work, the scientists who examined the long lasting effects of acupuncture as compared to exercise in women with PCOS, stated "Repeated EA treatments induce regular ovulations in more than one third of the women with PCOS." Further, for this group of women, electro-acupuncture (EA) can be an alternative to pharmacological ovulation induction.

I discourage my patients from asking whether diet, exercise or acupuncture works best. Each of these interventions can change the progression of PCOS, pregnancy, live birth rates and the varied health problems associated with this disease. Remember, both Western and OM PCOS treatment starts with loosing 5-10 lbs through improved diet and lifestyle. Unfortunately, this is often easier said than done. Some women, no matter how hard they try, insist that the scale will not budge! For these patients, I suggest keeping a food and exercise journal and if they haven't already, testing their thyroid. Most of the time, these two interventions nudge the scale downwards, but not always. For women who find diet and exercise to be insufficient, the addition of acupuncture can be the key to reaching their health and fertility goals. Research tells us that acupuncture can be used instead of diet or exercise modifications for weight reduction, hormonal regulation and ovulation induction. I don't recommend it. I do my best to impress upon my patients that all three of these factors work synergistically to induce lasting change.

Summing Up the Research

A literature review is a type of study where researchers evaluate as many studies as they can find on a central topic, pool the results and draw conclusions from the data. A comprehensive literature review including studies published on acupuncture and PCOS between 1970 and 2009, confirms what the Chinese have known for thousands of years. Researchers concluded that, "Acupuncture is a safe and effective treatment for PCOS".

Herbal Therapy for PCOS

While I was in China, I observed that women with PCOS received individualized herbal prescriptions based on their Chinese medical diagnosis. There were several different basic formulas used for PCOS, but as with acupuncture treatment, herbal therapy was tailored to the individual. Additionally, prescriptions changed during each phase of the menstrual cycle.

In PCOS, formulas that support yin and blood are given during the follicular phase. Care must be taken to make sure that while strengthening the yin, dampness doesn't accumulate. Remember, many women with PCOS tend towards excessive dampness, so herbs that promote circulation to the reproductive organs, nourish the ovaries AND discourage the accumulation of dampness are key to producing a good follicular phase and dominant follicle. During ovulation, the emphasis is on moving blood and qi to help a follicle break free from the ovary and move, unimpeded, down the fallopian tube.

The luteal phase herbal formulas for those with PCOS tend to emphasize strengthening the yang and promoting the receptivity of the womb for implantation. Because of the complex hormonal imbalances experienced by women with PCOS, the yin (follicular) phase may not be quite strong enough to support the yang (luteal). So, augmenting the yang while gently promoting circulation is a key principal in the herbal treatment of PCOS. In California, where licensed acupuncturist are able to order blood tests and prescribe herbal medicinals, ovulation can be monitored by the traditional methods of tongue and pulse reading, in addition to day 21 progesterone serum tests. And of course, most importantly, pregnancy rates!!!

There is a wealth of research on herbal treatments for different facets of PCOS. Cutting edge research on humans and animals suggests that precise, individualized herbal formulas can normalize insulin secretion, induce ovulation, regulate menstruation and normalize testosterone and LH/FSH levels. This research was conducted using ancient formulas from source texts as well as intramuscular injections of ginseng (something which the ancient Chinese simply couldn't do). An interesting outcome of the research on ginseng and PCOS was that researchers found that Korean red ginseng affected PCOS by suppressing the sympathetic nervous system's effect on the ovaries, thus allowing them greater blood flow, just like an acupuncture treatment!

The East: The Seat of Integrative Herbal and Western Medicine
It is interesting to note that in some parts of the world acupuncture, herbal formulas, and hormonal treatments are routinely used in conjunction with each other to promote fertility in PCOS patients. In my experience, the idea of combining herbal prescriptions with hormonal treatments makes most Western reproductive endocrinologists uneasy. In Japan and China, it's common practice. Several studies have compared and combined various herbal formulas to metformin, Clomid and gonadotropins in an effort to determine the best treatments for PCOS. In a paper published in the Chinese Journal of Integrated Medicine, scholars noted that it is common practice in China to combine Chinese and Western therapies for PCOS for the purpose of fertility enhancement.

O.K. It seems like there are a lot of options for me to pick from and even combine. But, I can't wait to get pregnant. So, I can go back to eating the mounds of bread, baked treats and candy that I love!

Remember, even after you conceive, diet and self-care are still important. You don't want to increase the chances of your girl developing PCOS, or your boy having deficits in sperm numbers and quality. The repercussions of what occurs while your child is developing in this environment could affect them during their reproductive years and beyond. And of course you want to minimize your risk of developing gestational diabetes.

OK, OK, but AFTER I deliver my healthy baby, THEN I can go back to eating the way I used to.

Of course you can. We all have the ability and the right to make choices that affect our bodies and our health. However, you should keep in mind that PCOS is more than just a fertility obstacle; it can affect every cell in your body.

Health Risks Associated With PCOS

- Insulin resistance, regardless of BMI
- Increased risk of type 2 diabetes
- Increased risk of heart disease
- Hypertension (high blood pressure)
- Endometrial cancer
- Impaired mental health

As you can see, not only can PCOS impair fertility, it can have lasting negative effects on your quality of life. **The good news is that you are NOT powerless!** You have several options in terms of fertility enhancement and regulation of your endocrine and metabolic systems. From diet and lifestyle changes, to Western and OM treatments, there IS help out there! I implore you to take this opportunity to learn about your body, enhance your fertility, and improve your quality of life, through your reproductive years and beyond.

Premature Ovarian Failure/Resistant Ovaries

According to Western medical theory, you were born with all of the eggs you will ever have (some OM practitioners disagree with this assertion). In the case of Premature Ovarian Syndrome (POF), the ovaries cannot, or when Resistant Ovary Syndrome (ROS) strikes, do not, respond to FSH. In both disorders, the outcome is infertility.

POF affects between 1-5% of women. It occurs when the ovaries stop functioning before age 40. In this situation, the pituitary is pumping out FSH in order to stimulate egg growth, but the ovary cannot respond. There simply are not enough follicles remaining. Fewer developing follicles results in low levels of estrogen. Essentially, women with POF have entered menopause at an early age.

Why does this happen?

POF is an enigma in Western medicine. There are several theories, but in about 2/3 of cases the underlying cause of POF is unknown. Speculations as to the root of POF include: autoimmune conditions, viral or bacterial infections and environmental toxins. We do know that there are genetic disorders that cause POF, such as Turner's syndrome and "fragile X syndrome". Cancer survivors may also develop POF as a consequence of radiation and chemotherapy.

ROS represents an even greater conundrum. In this condition there are plenty of follicles left, the ovary could mature and release a healthy egg…it just doesn't. Due to the lack of response from the ovaries, the pituitary puts out more and more FSH, which the ovaries ignore. As in POF, the explanation for why this happens is illusive. A virus, rendering the ovaries temporally unable to respond to FSH could be the culprit, or the ovaries could simply go through a phase of unresponsiveness for some other reason. Some women with ROS resume ovulation and go one to conceive, while others do not.

To understand these disorders better, let's take a look at the life cycle of an egg. Eggs originate deep inside the ovary in the form of primordial follicles. At this stage they do not have a direct blood supply, nor do they have FSH or other hormone receptors. They cannot be measured by ultrasounds, blood tests or other imaging tests. Primordial follicles are simply potential eggs. *If* all goes well, it takes 150 days for a primordial follicle to mature and ovulate.

So, if primordial follicles can't be measured and counted, how do I know how many I have left, or how healthy they are?

With current technology, you can't know without having your ovaries surgically removed, cut open and counting the potential eggs. However, chances are, that if you are reading this book, removing and damaging your ovaries is the last thing you want to do.

The maturation process of follicles to mature eggs goes something like this: primordial follicle -> primary follicle -> secondary follicle -> antral follicle -> dominant follicle -> ovulation. This development from primordial follicle to ovulation can take up to one year. This fact bears repeating. The egg you ovulated last month started developing one year ago. This means that it may take up to one year to truly know how you are going to respond to OM treatment. FSH only impacts the last 50 days of follicular development.

Unfortunately, Western medicine offers little assistance to women with POF and ROS. Drugs that stimulate the ovaries don't help, because the ovaries will not respond. However, OM treatment offers a different approach that encourages the resumption of ovulation and fertility by correcting underlying imbalances and restoring health. In OM theory, women with POF and ROS have a disruption in the Bao Mai or Bao Luo, causing anovulation. Treatment can be a long process, considering the lifespan of a follicle, and the fact that there's no good way to accurately measure your potential number of follicles. Fortunately, there are several points where OM treatment can impact follicular development. The length of time it may take for OM therapies to produce tangible results depends on which aspect of the year-long developmental process is being disrupted.

One factor I always consider when treating POF and ROS is environmental toxins that could be binding FSH receptors in the ovaries, rendering them unable to respond to endogenous FSH. Clinically, I've seen toxicity play a remarkable role in POF and ROS. Toxic heat can burn through the yin, jing, qi and blood, impairing the communication between the Uterus, Heart and Kidneys. Other potential OM patterns include: impaired Liver function, low Kidney energy, jing deficiency, and blood or qi stasis. The treatment and prognosis for each woman depends on the nuances of her OM diagnosis. These are difficult conditions to treat, but not impossible. OM treatment options all have one aspect in common - the side effect of increasing overall health.

Advanced Maternal Age

Your chronological age and your ovarian age may not be the same, as we saw in POF. But what is the normal physiology of reproductive aging in women? Interestingly, just as in OM, Western medicine views the years between ages 35 and 42 as critical, with rapidly decreasing fertility potential. Women can get pregnant during their early to mid-forties. However, keep in mind that as maternal age rises, pregnancy rates (both natural and assisted conception) go down, while the incidences of miscarriage and birth defects go up.

A key aspect of preserving fertility as we age is slowing down the aging cycles. We spoke in The Roots of Fertility chapter of: jing, yin, yang, qi, blood, prenatal essence and postnatal essence. You may also recall from this chapter, that while we were born with our prenatal (pre-heaven) essence in tact, we can change, for better or worse, our postnatal (post-heaven) essence. Postnatal essence can be increased by eating well, managing stress and by making positive lifestyle choices. If you generate more qi and blood than you use daily, they can nourish your prenatal essence and SLOW DOWN your aging cycle. If you use as much qi and blood as you make in a day, then you break even. If you are continuously using more energy than you produce, the aging process SPEEDS UP. So again, we encounter the OM concept that being as healthy as possible is an essential part of fertility enhancement for women *and men.*

My doctor said I have poor "ovarian reserve". How did that happen? What can I do to change this?

The affects of aging on ovaries include: scar tissue, decreased blood and oxygen supply, and increased damage to eggs due to free radical damage. This can cause both the quality and quantity of eggs to decline. As a result, older ovaries are less able to respond to FSH from the pituitary. So, the pituitary puts out more FSH. Typically, at first, estrogen levels rise and can become too high, too early in the cycle. Then, after a period of time, estrogen levels decrease as fewer follicles respond to the pituitary's signals and fertility declines. This process escalates until menopause, when the pituitary realizes that the ovaries are no longer going to react to FSH, so it stops emitting this hormone. Ovulation stops as does menstruation.

Thus, the easiest (though not the most accurate) measure of ovarian reserve is a FSH test. For this test, blood is drawn and FSH is measured on day three of your cycle. It's important to note that FSH levels can differ greatly from cycle to cycle and from lab to lab. This is important to keep in mind if you are comparing results from two different labs over a period of months. Ideally, your FSH should be six or under. Over six, but less than nine is pretty good. Between nine and twelve is not ideal. FSH over 15 is a red flag. Many fertility clinics will not perform IVF if your FSH is over 20. If your FSH is 12 one month, and 8 the next, this is a good sign. But you can't draw definite conclusions from these results. Many reproductive endocrinologists judge your fertility potential based on your highest FSH score.

Your fertility specialist may run additional blood tests to determine your "ovarian age". Anti-mullerian hormone (AMH) is secreted from the ovaries directly and does not fluctuate during the menstrual cycle. Therefore, this test may be used to gather information about the quantity, though not the quality of remaining eggs and can be done at any time during the month. Inhibin b is another hormone secreted by the ovary. This hormone acts on the pituitary and affects FSH levels. Some practitioners feel it can be helpful in determining egg quality and quantity.

Another test to determine how many eggs you have left is the Clomid Challenge Test. FSH is taken on day three and again after taking Clomid for 5 days in the beginning of your cycle. Both FSH measurements should be low. If not, it may indicate that you have fewer eggs left. While the day-three FSH and the Clomid Challenge tests are commonly used to determine ovarian potential, there is a theoretical problem with these tests. Remember, primordial follicles do not have FSH receptors. Only follicles that are very developed, within two months of maturation, have these hormone receptors. What if there were steps you could take to make your remaining follicles develop in such a way that they were more responsive to FSH? What if you could turn back the clock or at least preserve the fertility potential that you have now? If you are diagnosed with poor ovarian reserve, you have several options.

Possible Effects of Acupuncture, Herbal Formulas & Nutritional Supplementation

- Improve ovarian response to FSH and LH
- Increase ovarian blood flow
- Reduce free radical damage
- Protect oocyte DNA
- Improve oocyte maturation

Plus, it's important to keep in mind that ovarian reserve tests do not predict who will become pregnant. It is simply one method of measuring fertility potential. Despite the fact that we all age, you can impact your biological clock with OM therapies and by the food and lifestyle choices you make every day.

Immunologic Infertility

There are several different types of immune disorders that can impair fertility. These can afflict both men and women. For our purposes we will limit our discussion to two common immunologic causes of infertility, autoimmune thyroid disorders and antisperm antibodies.

What is autoimmunity?

A key part of an immune system is its ability to distinguish self from nonself. The immune system makes antibodies against and to attack viruses, bacteria and other potential threats. In autoimmune conditions, for reasons that are not fully understood, the immune system is triggered by parts of ourselves which are clearly not threats such as: organs, connective tissue, nerves, specific cells, hormones, neurotransmitters, etc.

Thyroid Autoimmunity (TAI)

We spoke earlier in this chapter about how important the thyroid gland is in menstrual regulation, fertility and fetal development. One of the most common autoimmune disorders in women of reproductive age is thyroid autoimmunity (TAI). TAI is an umbrella term that encompasses a range of thyroid autoimmune conditions such as antibodies to thyroid hormones and/or proteins within the thyroid. While TAI is one of the main causes of hyperthyroidism and hypothyroidism; this disorder can be present in women with normal thyroid function. Unfortunately, even in women with normal thyroid hormone levels, the presence of TAI can affect the ability to conceive and maintain a pregnancy. TAI is more likely to be found in women with other immune system imbalances such as endometriosis.

In Western medicine, the treatment for TAI is close monitoring of thyroid activity and thyroid hormone replacement if necessary. In OM the goal is to treat the underlying imbalance and restore normal immune function. Additionally, herbal formulas that modulate the immune system may also be prescribed. There have been several interesting studies on acupuncture's affect on autoimmune conditions.

Moxabustion and TAI

Scientists in Shanghai treated 71 people with TAI utilizing moxabustion and observed changes in immune and thyroid function. Interestingly, the amount of thyroid antibodies dropped and thyroid function normalized. Researchers believe that these effects were accomplished by moxabustion's ability to regulate white blood cell activity, specifically T lymphocytes.

Antisperm Antibodies (ASABs)

ASABs are found in up to 25% of couples struggling to conceive, as opposed to 2% of fertile couples. Both men and women can produce ASABs. In this situation, the man, the woman, or both, make antibodies to sperm. There are several reasons why this may occur. They include infection, testicular trauma or faulty barriers in the genital or digestive tracts or testicles that are supposed to keep the sperm separate from the blood steam. ASABs can bind to sperm even before ejaculation, rendering them less motile. Fertilization rates can be reduced by 80% when the cervix and fallopian tubes secrete ASABs.

Western treatments for this condition include: a barrier method of birth control and steroids. Some physicians advocate using a condom for several months then resume trying to conceive. Men may also be prescribed a controversial treatment consisting of high doses of steroids to reduce inflammation and suppress the immune system. This therapy can last for 9 months or more. Unfortunately, the efficacy of this treatment is questionable and long-term use of steroids can cause many side effects such as bone and joint weakening and erosion.

Not only can ASABs affect natural conception rates, they also reduce the effectiveness of assisted reproductive techniques. Intra-uterine insemination (IUI) success rates are low in cases of high ASABs, in part because antibodies cannot be removed from the sperm without causing them significant damage. IVF with assisted fertilization where sperm are injected directly into an egg (ICSI) is often the best Western fertility treatment for these patients. Detailed information on IVF, IUI and ICSI is presented in the Assisted Reproductive Techniques (ART) chapter.

How can OM help couples with ASABs?

In both men and women ASABs commonly present as toxic heat, blood stasis and kidney yin deficiency. Only recently have we had the technology to view ASABs. However, studies in China have demonstrated that acupuncture and ancient herbal fertility promoting formulas can reduce ASABs and increase pregnancy rates.

Treating ASABs—East Vs. West

Several research studies have demonstrated Chinese medicine to be very successful in treating ASABs in both men and women. In one of these studies, 100 men with ASABs were divided into two groups. One group received acupuncture and herbal therapy while the other was treated with steroids. Both groups showed a significant decline in ASABs, 90% for the Chinese medicine treated group and 64% for the steroid treated group. The authors of this study reported that acupuncture and Chinese herbal treatment was superior to Western drug treatment due to the significantly higher response of the acupuncture group without the side effects associated with steroid treatment.

Unexplained Infertility/Subfertility

Unexplained infertility is the diagnosis reached after ruling out all other factors that can cause infertility. If, after undergoing a barrage of tests to measure hormone and antibody levels, imaging tests, one or more semen analyses and possibly exploratory surgery, no obvious cause for lack of conception can be found, a couple faces the label of unexplained infertility.

The Western treatment for unexplained infertility consists of a combination of hormones to boost egg production and ovulation, coupled with techniques to encourage fertilization. Clomid with or without Intra-Uterine-Insemination (IUI) is typically the first line of treatment in cases of unexplained infertility. This is because this procedure is the least expensive and invasive treatment in comparison to other forms of artificial reproductive techniques (ART). This treatment offers an overall success rate of approximately 8%. Typically, three to four of these cycles are performed successively before changing treatment modalities. Evidence indicates that women with unexplained infertility may have a lower uterine blood supply in the follicular phase. Ironically, taking Clomid may worsen the situation by reducing blood flow to the uterus during the periimplantion stage, thus reducing uterine lining thickness. Given the low success rate of Clomid and IUI, some couples opt to go directly to IVF.

I was just diagnosed with unexplained infertility. Is there anything I can do to increase my chances of natural conception?

Absolutely. Perhaps a better name for "unexplained infertility" is subfertility. Degrees of subfertility vary between partners. However, it is estimated that between 30-50% of couples are subfertile. This represents a hurdle towards pregnancy but not a complete barrier. A very common picture in clinical practice is as follows: A 39 year old male's sperm count is 20 million, which today is considered normal, but historically would be low. His partner is 34. Her periods are regularly spaced, but she has pain with ovulation and some breakthrough bleeding (bleeding in the middle of a cycle). This couple could very well receive an "unexplained infertility" diagnosis, when in fact they are simply subfertile. He could use help improving his sperm count, while she could benefit by improving her menstrual cycle.

Herbal Formulas Can Help Couples with Unexplained Infertility
In London, researchers measured the effects of Chinese herbal formulas on several markers of female fertility. These markers were measured before the study and again after treatment with Chinese herbs. The herbal formulas were specifically tailored to each individual woman's OM diagnosis. Six months after the conclusion of the study, researchers counted a total of 28 women out of 50 who fell pregnant. Just think of how many more pregnancies could have been achieved if the men were treated too!

Miscarriage
By definition, those who have suffered a miscarriage are not infertile. Still, up to one third of these couples likely faced fertility challenges before conceiving. It can be easy for fertility specialists and prospective parents to place such emphasis on getting pregnant, that they loose perspective of what is most important: delivering a healthy baby. It is imperative to keep that ultimate goal in mind. The holistic OM view of fertility includes not only a confirmed pregnancy, but a healthy pregnancy,

smooth delivery and parents with the energy and stamina to take care of a newborn baby. These steps can all be influenced before conception by bolstering the health of the prospective mother and father. Improvements in these areas sets the stage for a healthy sperm and egg to unite, a plush environment for implantation and the foundation for a strong pregnancy.

Becky's Story

When Becky, a 38 year old woman, called my office, she was 10 weeks pregnant. However, that morning an ultrasound failed to detect a fetal heart beat and it appeared the fetus had stopped growing at 8 weeks. The baby had died, but Becky's body had yet to go into a mini labor, i.e. a miscarriage. Her OB/GYN wanted her to undergo a dilation and curettage (D&C). This procedure cleans the womb and removes the products of conception. Becky didn't want to do an invasive procedure, she wanted her body to "do what it is supposed to" and miscarry naturally. Becky had never tried acupuncture before, but wanted to know if acupuncture could naturally induce a miscarriage.

I told Becky that I understood how she felt; that undergoing a surgical technique to accomplish what her body should naturally do on its own did not feel right to her. I also suggested she go through with the D&C. While strong manipulation of specific acupuncture points can cause miscarriage, it is not commonly practiced in the United States because of the risk of incomplete miscarriage, which can result in infection or hemorrhage.

While I suggested she follow the Western route first, I emphasized the benefit acupuncture and herbal formulas to nourish her depleted qi and blood, regulate her hormones and prepare her for another pregnancy.

Becky and I worked together for several months until she felt secure in her health and was ready to try again. She conceived during her first month of trying and is now mother to a healthy baby boy.

How common are miscarriages?

It is difficult to estimate, but a commonly accepted statistic is 20% of pregnancies miscarry. There are several different causes for this. While miscarriages can occur at any point in pregnancy, most miscarriages happen within the first trimester and are often the result of fetal genetic abnormalities or maternal hormone imbalances. For example, as we discussed previously, thyroid problems can cause infertility and result in miscarriages. Italian researchers followed over 4000 pregnant women to determine what impact TSH had on miscarriage rates. They found that while hypo and hyperthyroidism and TAI all had adverse effects on pregnancy outcome, TSH levels over 2.5, previously considered normal, can dramatically increase miscarriage rates.

There is also a strong relationship between the age of the potential parents and incidence of miscarriage. The older a woman is when she conceives, the more likely she is to miscarry. While the overall chance of miscarriage is 16% for women under the age of 35, those rates rise dramatically to 50% or more when a woman reaches the age of 46. While the relationship between a woman's age and the odds of miscarriage is common knowledge among medical practitioners, research now suggests that her partner's age also impacts miscarriage rates. In women over 35, the effects of her partner's age on conception and miscarriage were masked, but younger women with partners over the age of 35 are twice as likely to miscarry than their counterparts with younger husbands.

It is estimated that only one in four fertilizations will result in a full term pregnancy. Sometimes the embryo never implants. If after sperm and egg unification the embryo does implant, it should start producing human chorionic gonadotropin (HCG), telling the ovary to keep producing progesterone. HCG is the hormone that blood and urine pregnancy tests are designed to detect.

Factors That Can Impede Pregnancy & Contribute to Miscarriage

- Endocrine abnormalities
- Exposure to toxins or x-rays
- Trauma
- Infection
- Endocrine abnormalities
- Immunological/Autoimmune disorders
- Hemolytic diseases
- Cervical or uterine structural anomalies
- Alcohol, smoking, drug use
- Endometriosis
- PCOS
- Advanced parental age
- Sperm abnormalities
- Luteal Phase Defect

Chinese Researchers Tackle Luteal Phase Defect

Put simply, a Luteal Phase Defect diagnosis implies that there is not enough progesterone present in the luteal phase of the cycle to create a lush uterine lining or sustain a pregnancy. Researchers in Nanjing studied sixty women with Luteal Phase Defect.

Subjects were treated with herbal formulas traditionally used to strengthen the kidneys, regulate qi and blood, and balance yin and yang. Study participants experienced stronger ovulations and increased luteal phase temperatures as evidenced by BBT charts. Of the sixty study participants, 32 fell pregnant.

I've already had one miscarriage, are there any simple/basic precautions I can take to prevent another?

Yes. If you smoke, drink or use drugs, stop. Get an annual exam to rule out common vaginal infections such as yeast and bacterial vaginosis. Eat a fertility friendly diet and minimize exposure to toxins. Some inexpensive lab tests can be very valuable. They should include a thyroid panel to make sure your thyroid is functioning OPTIMALLY, including: TSH, fT3, fT4, TPO and reverse T3. Female hormone panels which include progesterone, FSH, LH, estrogen, testosterone, and progesterone are important. Markers of immune function and inflammation should be evaluated; such as antiphospholipid antibodies and homocystine levels, especially in women who have a history of miscarriage. I prefer to work in conjunction with a reproductive endocrinologist (RE) when my patient has had two or more serial miscarriages. An RE can facilitate genetic testing or imaging studies when necessary. According to research, the timing of intercourse can impact the chances of pregnancy loss in women who have experienced a miscarriage. The best time for these couples to have intercourse is the day before ovulation or the day of ovulation.

While incidences of miscarriage are relatively common, the good news is that the number of couples that face recurrent miscarriage is small, between 1-3%. Recurrent miscarriage is defined as three or more miscarriages within a relationship. This syndrome can be heartbreaking for couples, as many of them have also faced fertility challenges. At this point, in-depth investigation is warranted, including analyzing the fetus for chromosomal defects and examining the parents for genetic abnormalities, as well as endocrine, anatomical and immune conditions.

Fertility Diet & Lifestyle

YOU CAN MAKE A huge impact on your fertility by adopting a fertility friendly diet and lifestyle. Quit smoking, give up that morning and afternoon coffee, pass on the glass or two of wine with dinner (and dessert) to shift your diet away from the Standard American Diet (SAD) to a pro-fertility one. Benefits include better overall health, reduced chance of chronic disease, and an increased chance of children! *The key to successfully altering your diet is keeping the right perspective. You're not depriving yourself of anything; you're giving yourself a better chance of conception.*

The suggestions in this chapter are for guys too! Couples have the opportunity to view this diet as a cleanse in which you both work towards the common goals of pregnancy and better health. Remember, this is a medicinal diet and lifestyle to help you achieve your goal. So, when you face challenges, like getting in your daily exercise, or choosing what you *can* eat in place of a donut, remind yourself that you made a choice to live in a way that cultivates life.

The East/West Fertility Diet

Six to twelve months of healthy living can make a huge impact on your quality of life and fertility potential. Inherent in a healthy living lifestyle are proper diet, exercise and stress management. Remember in earlier chapters when we talked about prenatal and postnatal essence? Prenatal essence is the potential you came into the world with, while postnatal essence is what you produce on a daily basis. You can use your postnatal essence to either supplement your prenatal essence, or drain it, depending on your daily behaviors. For a refresher in OM theory and its perspective on fertility, see The Roots of Fertility chapter. Suffice it to say that optimizing your fertility requires an abundance of postnatal essence. Not only what, but also HOW you eat, drink and exercise can help you towards your goal of bursting at the seams with postnatal essence. Some of the following Chinese dietary guidelines may sound strange and conflict with conventional ideas about healthy eating, but these principals are time tested and true. Many of them have been confirmed by a Harvard Nurses' Study, so keep an open mind as you read on.

Wisdom From the East

Hot & Cold- Cooked foods are better than raw foods. Lightly steaming your broccoli and cooked spinach salads are better choices than their raw counterparts. The Chinese are not big fans of salads. I know, this goes against everything you have ever heard about healthy eating. This is a general OM dietary principal. While some people do OK with cold, raw foods, most of us do not. In my experience, younger men tend to do better than women with a raw food diet. According to OM theory, women trying to conceive should pass up salads for soups and opt for steamed or lightly sautéed veggies instead of raw ones.

I've seen this subject bring people to tears. "But I love my salads!" and "How am I going to loose weight if I don't eat salads!?" I've found that often people don't necessarily love their salads per se; they love that they don't feel stuffed and sluggish after eating. This could be from what they are *not* eating, rather than what they *are* eating. For example, perhaps you're having a salad instead of a burger and fries. Yes, a burger and fries is a hot meal, but common sense tells us that given a choice between grease (often served with a soda) and salad, many people will feel better after a salad. But what if you could feel good after eating foods that are fertility friendly AND taste good. That burger may still be on the menu after all, just not the fries, soda or ice water.

At restaurants, ask for your water without ice. Drinks should be room temperature – the exception being if you are in very hot weather - but even then, go easy on the frozen drinks.

But what about smoothies?

Yes, I know. Smoothies are supposed to rank high in terms of their health benefits. You can make wonderfully healthy smoothies; just leave out the frozen fruit and ice. In fact, if you're a fruit junkie, you should cut way down on the fruit. We'll talk more about that later in this chapter.

Meat & Fish - If you are vegetarian, can you incorporate some meat? If you are vegan, can you add in eggs and milk? Remember, these would be changes for medicinal purposes. Vegetarianism isn't part of a traditional OM diet. The concept of vegetarianism doesn't make sense to most of the Chinese physicians with whom I have discussed this subject. As a country with a history filled with famine, animals are to be eaten modestly, and not taken for granted. Animals such as chickens and cows have taken nutrients from plants and converted it into essence and blood. Thus using animal parts for medicinal purposes has a long history in China. As far as I know, animals intended for consumption were fed a vegetarian diet, not given antibiotics or growth hormones, nor were they brought in from distant lands. Therefore, animals from which we get eggs, milk and meat should be vegetarian/grass fed, free range, local and organic. This principal goes for vegetables and fruits too. Local, seasonal foods should make up the bulk of your diet. If you're unwilling to incorporate animal products into your diet, you can still eat to conceive. Simply bear in mind the principals behind eating animals (i.e. deep nourishment) and do your best to build your diet around this idea.

Nourishing Prenatal Essence- There are specific foods known to boost prenatal essence such as nuts, seeds and eggs. Fresh raw nuts that are not roasted and salted are best. For most people, nuts other than peanuts (which are not really nuts) are better. Peanuts can cause inflammation. For example, walnuts are a good option because of their plentiful anti-inflammatory omega oils. Almonds are also a good choice for nourishing your yin. Simply soak your almonds in water for a few hours before eating. Flax seeds are rich in omega oils, but when ground, go rancid very quickly. Keep flax seeds and flax oil in the freezer. Cooking with flax oil will destroy its anti-inflammatory benefits. Add ground flax seeds or flax oil to dishes for a flavor boost. Macadamia nut oil is another anti-inflammatory flavor enhancer, but should only be used for very low heat cooking. Many oils are sensitive to heat and go rancid at high temperatures. Use olive oil for medium heat cooking and canola for higher heat. Store your olive oil in the refrigerator. Eggs are a potent source of protein. In many health food stores you can find omega-3 eggs, which come from chickens fed vegetarian diets high in flax seeds.

Mindful Eating

Do you eat on the go? Do you use the cup holders in your car for your daily coffee? Do you nibble on the donut or scone in the other cup holder next to your coffee on the freeway or at stoplights on your way to work? How about lunch? Is it a cold salad with a soda at your desk while working, or is it fast food? Do you chew quietly on fries during a phone call with clients or colleagues during your lunch break? At about 3:30 in the afternoon do you have a coffee with sugar bomb disguised as a "healthy pumpkin muffin" from the nearby coffee shop? Tired yet? By the time you get off work, you are dragging and can't imagine making dinner. So, it's fast food, right? If others depend on you to prepare dinner, maybe it's a frozen pizza, spaghetti, or some other food that comes out of a box and only requires water and heat? Oh, and don't forget dessert! Ice cream, cookies, brownies, what ever you like, because you deserve it. You've had a hard day. Add a glass or two of wine to "calm down" from the day and it's off to bed with restless sleep so you can do it all over again tomorrow.

Sound Familiar?

For most Americans, this is a typical routine. Switch pretzels or candy for the pumpkin muffin and it's basically the same. We know that there are several components of this diet that need to change. But notice that it's not just *what* we're eating, it's also *how* we're eating. The Chinese contend that a healthy digestive system and nutritious meal begins with a calm environment. This principal applies to men and women. We have talked in prior chapters about the two parts of the autonomic nervous system. The parasympathetic helps you eat, digest, relax, and sleep. The sympathetic is activated in times of stress. The body doesn't want to digest food if it thinks it may have to run from a tiger. While your boss may not look like a tiger, your body experiences both forms of stress in a very primitive way called "fight or flight". We either need to defend ourselves from the tiger (or our boss), or run away to fight another day. Working at lunch or speeding to work in the morning stirs up a physiological response you needed thousands of years ago to stay alive. But, constant triggering of the sympathetic nervous system can make you feel both tired *and* "wired". You certainly can't digest food properly under these conditions. What good is the best diet in the world if you can't digest it?

Living in a predominantly sympathetic mode reduces your ability to conceive for two reasons:

1. It directs blood and energy away from the reproductive system.
2. The endocrine system prioritizes making stress hormones over those necessary for fertility.

Listed are a few tricks to shift this pattern, which will also make other dietary improvements easier to accomplish:

- *Chew your food!* Sound like your Mom? Well, Mom was on to something. Your digestive enzymes start to work on food as you chew. Plus, chewing is your first defense against aflatoxins. These toxins are produced by mold that commonly grows on nuts, seeds, grains, and beans. Aflatoxins are carcinogenic and NOT fertility friendly. In addition to chewing your food, adding carrots, parsnips, celery, parsley, dill and other members of the apiaceous vegetable family will help you counteract aflatoxins.
- *Eat peacefully.* Don't discuss politics over a meal. Don't read the newspaper or work while eating. If you have an important business lunch appointment, eat beforehand. That way you can spend your time discussing issues, as opposed to talking with your mouth full.
- *A short walk after eating* will help your body balance its blood sugar levels and give you an opportunity to walk off some stress.
- *Eat several small meals* throughout the day and STOP *before* you are full. Eat slowly and use a small plate. These habits are easier to incorporate in your life

than it may sound. Eat half of what you would normally eat for lunch, and then take a short walk. If you don't work in an environment that is conducive to walking, just walk up and down the stairs in your building a few times. Twenty minutes after your last bite, if you're still hungry, finish your lunch. If you're not hungry, remind yourself that you can eat more at any time. Put your food away and eat more of it a couple of hours later. I'd be willing to bet that you'll be surprised by how much more food you consume than you actually need.

- *Cutting down on your calories* can actually give you more energy. Coupled with changing how you eat, you may be joyfully surprised by the feedback from your scale after just a few weeks!

Wisdom From the West

While Western medicine can't give us thousands of years of empirically tested fertility guidelines, it does provide us with research on how weight and specific nutrients affect fertility.

What is Your Target Fertility Weight? Your Body Mass Index (BMI)

When I was growing up, the commonly held belief for calculating your proper weight was as follows: at 5 ft tall, you should weigh 100 lbs. Add 5 lbs for every inch taller than 5 ft. So, if you were 5'9", your weight should hover around 145 lbs. This is an easy to calculate method that you can do in your head to estimate what your weight "should be". For a more precise gauge of your ideal weight, and where you fall on the underweight to obese continuum, calculate your BMI. People often ask me how to do that, as it's not easy to calculate in your head. This is why we have calculators and computers!

Your BMI = Your Weight in lbs. multiplied by 703, divided by your height in inches, divided by your height in inches again. So our 5'9" woman who weighs 145 lbs. has a BMI of 21.4. Her weight (145 lbs.) multiplied by 703= 101935 / height in inches (69) = is 1477.3188405797101 / height in inches again (69) = 21.410417979416089, or simply 21.4. Did I mention that this isn't something most people can do in their heads? So, grab a calculator or visit: nhlbisupport.com/bmi/mbinojs.htm

What can my BMI tell me?

This is a very important question. The ranges of BMI measurements are as follows: 18.5 and under is considered underweight, between 19 and 25 is normal, between 25 and 30 is overweight, and over 30 is obese. If you are a very muscular person, keep in mind that muscle weighs more than fat. Thus, people with regular exercise routines may have higher BMIs, but that doesn't make them overweight. This is important to remember when evaluating your target fertility weight.

The Harvard Nurses' Study

In 1976, scientists from the Harvard School of Public Health began one of the largest and longest studies on record. This study came to be known as "The Harvard Nurses' Study". Over 200,000 women answered detailed questions about their diet, behaviors and lives. Analyzing data over decades, researchers found trends between diet, weight, and anovulatory infertility. Women with BMIs between 20-24 were less likely to suffer from anovulatory infertility. Those who ate a whole grain diet with plentiful protein from vegetable sources, exercised, emphasized monounsaturated fats, took a multivitamin, and had a small amount of full fat dairy every day were less likely to suffer from this type of infertility as well. The Harvard Nurses' Study has changed the way we think about diet, weight and fertility.

Building Blocks of the Fertility Diet: Carbohydrates

Once upon a time, common wisdom held that carbohydrates should make up the bulk of a healthy diet. It didn't matter what kind of carbohydrate it was, bread, rice, sugar, fruit, or vegetables, the body treated them all the same. It was also believed that fat used in making food was the culprit in weight gain. By this reasoning, if you stayed away from fat, you wouldn't get fat.

Well, these ideas didn't work. We have grown heavier as a nation in spite of the low-fat/high-carbohydrate food craze. Over the last decade, carbohydrates have earned a bad reputation. The latest diet trends denounce carbs and emphasize fats and protein. However, the Harvard Nurses' Study tells us that this isn't the whole picture.

Carbohydrates are a necessary nutrient group. They give us energy. However, not all carbohydrates are metabolized equally. Slow burning carbohydrates are good for fertility, while quickly digestible carbohydrates can spike insulin and blood sugar levels, disrupting the delicate hormonal balance needed for ovulation and a healthy pregnancy. The Harvard Nurses' Study demonstrated that the quality of carbohydrate intake is more important than the quantity.

The "Good" Carbs

- Whole Grains (unprocessed oats, brown rice, wild rice, quinoa, millet, etc.)
- Vegetables
- Legumes (beans are also wonderful sources of protein)

The "Bad" Carbs

- Processed flour products (white bread, scones, white pasta, bagels and chips, etc.)
- Candy, cookies, brownies, cake, ice cream
- French fries, pizza
- Soda, alcohol, sugary drinks (ex: chai with honey or sugar)

But what about the glycemic index? It seems I'm always hearing that term used to describe good and bad food. What is it and how does it fit in?

The glycemic index (GI) is a comparison of how foods act in the body. It was developed by scientists who measured the ability of different foods to act like pure glucose in the body, triggering insulin release and acting on the body's blood sugar levels. In this system, foods are divided into low, medium and high GI. Foods in the low and middle categories are generally better for your blood sugar balance than high GI foods. While the GI is helpful, it's not the whole story. For example, fructose (the sugar in fruit) barely registers on the GI, because the liver takes on the brunt of processing it. Some foods, like carrots, have a very high GI, but when typical servings are taken into account, the practical impact on blood sugar decreases. This measurement is called the glycemic load (GL). Sound complicated?

Calculating the GL on the go isn't so hard if you remember a few simple rules:

1. Remember that fruit is nature's sugar. Go easy on fruit. Stay away from fruit juice, which has the fiber stripped out (at best) and sugar added (at worst).
2. The more fiber a food has, the better. Fiber slows the body's blood sugar response. As a rule of thumb, don't eat "anything white", potatoes, white rice, white bread, white pasta, etc. Choose their whole grain counterparts, yams and sweet potatoes.
3. Experiment with grains. There is a wide world of whole grains out there beyond rice. Try amaranth, millet or quinoa. If this sounds a little too foreign at the moment, get started by experimenting with different types of rice like wild or brown.
4. It's best to have a protein or good fat with your carbohydrate. Don't just eat whole grain pasta with butter—add sauce with lean meat or textured vegetable protein or mix the pasta with a good fat like olive oil, with a serving of salmon

on the side. Add these to your meal to bring down the GI: cinnamon, lemon juice and vinegar.

5. When in doubt, look it up. For the GI of almost 1,600 foods, visit: www.glycemicindex.com.

Wow, I have a huge sweet tooth. How can I possibly give up my sweets?

You don't have to. Commit to two weeks of sugar abstinence. As you decrease the amount of high fructose corn syrup, cane sugar and other sweets, a whole new world will open up to you. Foods that you never thought were sweet before, because your taste buds were over-stimulated, now have the opportunity to shine through as you become much more sensitive to sweet tastes. Plus, while there's conflicting evidence regarding the long-term safety of many sugar substitutes, there is also some interesting data suggesting that a certain type of sugar replacement may be more than just OK for you.

What could be better than sugar?

Sugar Polyols are carbohydrates, used as sugar replacements, that taste sweet but are not absorbed. Researchers examined the benefits of several different types of sugar polyols such as: xylitol, sorbitol, mannitol, and maltitol, among others. They found, on the whole, that these sugar polyols won't give you cavities or cause your blood sugar to spike. What's more, they can regulate the micro flora of the intestines.

However, note that sugar polyols are used to treat constipation. In sensitive individuals they can cause gas, bloating and diarrhea. Additionally, just because you buy candy with this sweetener doesn't mean it's low in calories. So, start small. Try one piece of candy to see how you tolerate it.

Many of these sugar polyols can be found in candy marketed to diabetics, or labeled as "diabetic safe candy". You may even find xylitol in the baking section of your local health food store. Xylitol is about as sweet as cane sugar, so when substituting it in your baking (with whole grain flour and good fats of course) use a 1:1 ratio. For example if your recipe calls for 1 cup of sugar, substitute 1 cup of xylitol.

Believe it or not, you can make delicious baked goods with sugar polyols. One of my patients, in an effort to reduce her inflammation, muscle and joint pain, switched from cane sugar to xylitol in her baking. By listening to her body's feedback, following OM dietary principals, and focusing on low GI foods, she drastically reduced her pain. OM and dietary therapy helped her accomplish her health goals with greater efficacy than any other Western or "alternative" therapy.

Meredith's Sugar-Free Lavender Coconut Mini Muffin Recipe

- **Preheat oven to 400F degrees:**

- **Mix together**
- ¼ teaspoon salt
- ½ cup coconut flour
- ½ cup almond flour
- ¼ teaspoon baking powder
- ½ teaspoon baking soda
- ½ cup unsweetened coconut flakes
- ⅛ teaspoon xanthum gum (but is not necessary)

- **Melt together over low heat**
- 1 stick butter (or 4 tablespoons coconut butter)
- ½ to ¾ cup xylitol (depending on how sweet you want it)
- 2 tablespoons lavender

- Melt butter on low heat. Add xylitol first and then lavender at the last minute.

- **Next mix together:**
- 1 egg
- 1 cup full fat raw milk
- 1 teaspoon vanilla extract

- Mix together dry ingredients, and then add all the wet ingredients including the mixed xylitol and lavender mixture. Consistency should be similar to a brownie mix, not runny, but not very firm.
- You can use mini muffin tins or large muffin tins. Mini is more fun for bite-sized treats! Grease the mini muffin tins or use muffin liners.
- Makes about 22 mini muffins
- Bake for 9 - 12 minutes or until a toothpick comes out clean and the tops are slightly golden. Enjoy!

Building Blocks of the Fertility Diet: Fats

As I mentioned earlier, fats don't deserve the bad reputation they gained in the 1980's. Some fats can actually help you LOSE weight. You need fat. Your body uses it for energy storage, to make hormones, to protect nerves, etc. Fats can help you feel satiated for longer, bring down the GI of a meal and exert anti-inflammatory effects. Some fats are anti-inflammatory, while others tend to be inflammatory. It all depends on what type of fat you are consuming: monounsaturated fats, polyunsaturated fats, saturated fats or trans fats.

Add monounsaturated and polyunsaturated fats to your diet. These fats come from nuts, vegetables, beans and fish. Yummy examples of these fats are: olives and olive oil, safflower oil, canola oil, flax seed oil, soybeans and soybean oil, salmon, herring, avocados, nuts, seeds and butters made from them - like pumpkin and sesame seed butters, almond, cashew and macadamia nut butters, etc. According to data gathered from the Harvard Nurses' Study, these fats boost fertility. They also have additional benefits such as regulating cholesterol, lowering inflammation and modulating blood sugar.

Focus on eating less saturated fat. Saturated fats are solid at room temperature. Butter is a saturated fat. The fat on your plate after you eat bacon is another example of saturated fat, as is milk fat, cheese and lard. While most saturated fats come from animals, some vegetable sources do exist. Coconut butter, coconut milk and coconut oil are examples of saturated fats that occur in nature. Coconut oil has been reported to help regulate blood sugar and improve calcium and magnesium absorption. While those are positive effects of coconut oil, on the whole, saturated fats are regarded as having a negative impact on fertility and may promote heart disease. So, eat them in strict moderation.

You should avoid trans fats completely. While saturated, monounsaturated and polyunsaturated fats are found in nature, the majority of trans fats in our food supply are the by-products of vegetable oil stabilization (to prevent rancidity). Only a small amount is present in dairy and meat. These fats are BAD for fertility and have negative effects on cardiovascular health. Trans fats are found in ready-made baked goods like cookies, fast food and restaurant fried foods. Consumption of these fats can decrease your chances of getting pregnant. There is evidence that they also increase your risk of cardiovascular disease, upset blood sugar levels and are likely to promote inflammation. The data from the Harvard Nurses' Study shows us that even moderate intake of trans fats can have negative effects on ovulation. How much is a moderate dose of trans fats? Only one doughnut or two tablespoons of margarine per day. The evidence is clear. Stay away from trans fats.

Building Blocks of the Fertility Diet: Protein

We Americans like our animal protein. As a nation, we eat almost 8 times more beef than we do beans. According to the Harvard Nurses' Study, following this trend may increase your risk of anovulatory infertility. Protein comes from many sources, the most well known to us are animals like beef, chicken and pork. Fish, beans and nuts also provide protein. Like fats and carbohydrates, we need protein, AND like fats and carbohydrates, the source of the nutrient can make the difference between eating for one and eating for two. Women in the Harvard Nurses' Study who tended to consume their protein from animal sources, were more likely to suffer from anovulatory infertility. Those with diets rich in vegetable sources of protein were much less likely to have this problem.

I've heard a lot of different opinions about protein. My nutritionist said I could damage my kidneys from eating too much. How much is too much, or too little?

This is the million-dollar question. Current wisdom holds that for someone weighing 140lbs it takes about 50 grams of protein per day to keep the body functioning smoothly. To find out how much protein you require, add 7 grams of protein for every 20lbs of weight. However, the amount of protein required to function and the target amount of protein for someone looking to become pregnant could be two different numbers. In my experience, it's unlikely that you'll get too much protein if you concentrate on the sources of protein. So, don't focus too much on the numbers. For example, unless you have kidney disease or osteoporosis, you can safely have 125 grams of protein per day (based on a 2,000 calorie diet). Adequate dietary protein can help you curb sugar cravings, keep you from feeling hungry longer after eating, and perhaps help you lose weight. Pay close attention to where you get your protein.

Focus On

- Beans
- Nuts
- Organic, free-range, animal products (such as a skinless chicken breast, one serving of full fat dairy or a little butter)
- Organic, free-range, grass fed, lean cuts of beef
- Organic, free-range, omega 3 enriched eggs
- Protein powders made from almond, pea, rice and hemp sources
- Nut milks like soy, hemp, almond, (with no sugar added) etc.
- Fish*

* Fish can be a wonderful source of protein and important omega 3 fatty acids like docosahexaenoic acid (a primary structural component of sperm and testicles). Unfortunately, fish can also be contaminated with mercury, dioxins and polychlorinated biphenyls (PCBs). Eating fish lower on the food chain tends to be safer. Go for sardines, wild salmon and trout. You can check the Environmental Defense Fund website, www.edf.org, for information about responsible and safe fish choices.

Suggestions For Specific Conditions

Women over the age of 35 may not ovulate each cycle, may ovulate early in their cycle or may produce poor quality eggs. Those with POF and ROS have difficulty ovulating at all, and those with PCOS generally ovulate infrequently.

Women over 35 and those with PCOS may produce eggs with harder shells that are difficult for sperm to penetrate. When I see women with these types of ovulatory dysfunction, I strongly encourage their partners to come in for treatment - even if his semen analysis is "O.K." His sperm need to be better than O.K. because they likely must penetrate a harder shell. We'll discuss male fertility enhancement in the next chapter. Suffice it to say, that this is an important and often overlooked component in helping couples with ovulatory disorders conceive.

In the Roots of Fertility chapter, we discussed how eggs mature within the ovary and the roles of prenatal and postnatal influences in egg development. You may not see an immediate payoff from working with your ovaries. This is important to keep in mind. To slow ovarian aging and nourish the eggs we have, the best strategy is to use postnatal essence (what this chapter is all about) to nourish prenatal essence.

This Is An Important Concept

- You can improve your fertility by using postnatal essence to nourish prenatal essence. So, if you have more energy from eating well, use it to strengthen your reproductive organs! **DO NOT USE IT UP BY STAYING AWAKE ALL NIGHT WORKING.**
- Unlike women with PCOS, those with POF, ROS and potentially women over 35, may have fewer eggs developing per month (in PCOS, there are several developing eggs, but an insufficient amount that mature). We have to ask ourselves, are the eggs stuck in the ovaries? Are there plenty of eggs and they're just not responding to FSH? If so, you may need to concentrate on ridding your system of EDCs, as they can bind to FSH receptors and disturb the process of egg maturation.
- Focus on reducing oxidative damage and inflammation. To this end, first be sure to get adequate vitamin D. You may need to get a vitamin D3 blood test from your primary care provider. In addition to a prenatal vitamin, you may want to take an antioxidant formula with plenty of D3, vitamin E and A (from beta-carotene), alpha lipoic acid (ALA), N-Acetal-Cystine (NAC), and B vitamins including folate, magnesium and chromium. When taken with meals, this can provide you with protection against oxidative damage and encourage healthy blood sugar metabolism. In women over 35 and those with PCOS, NAC may be useful as it can reduce the thickness of the egg's shell.

PCOS

FOLLOW THE EAST/WEST FERTILITY DIET! Remember, the Western contribution to this diet comes from a study that followed women with ANOVULATORY infertility. While not exactly synonymous with PCOS, anovulation is a major symptom of PCOS and of significant concern to women trying to become pregnant. While many women with PCOS are overweight, or at least not underweight, there are PCOS patients who struggle to keep weight on. I have treated women with PCOS who find it difficult not to lose weight, even though they have athocanthus nigrans (a darkening of the skin due to insulin resistance). These patients require care above and beyond the dietary guidelines described in this chapter. I've found acupuncture and herbal formulas to be essential for these patients. Overweight women may jump start the endocrine system and monthly ovulation by simply dropping 10 lbs.

How can I lose that weight?

Add exercise to your daily routine. A 20-minute brisk walk per day counts - if you break a sweat. Embrace a low GI diet. Don't eat foods that can spike your blood sugar such as white rice, potatoes, chips, crackers, bread, scones, bagels and other baked goods. You may not even be able to eat whole grains daily or you may need to limit your fruit intake (though these changes should only be made under the supervision of a qualified health care provider). You should see signs of improvement, such as a reduction in one or all of your PCOS symptoms. If you don't drop at least 5 lbs after two months of rigorously following the East/West Fertility Diet, consult a health care provider familiar with the Paleo diet and other blood sugar regulatory diets.

Modulating Inflammation and the Immune System

Women who struggle with autoimmune disease such as thyroiditis (and some argue that endometriosis is also autoimmune in nature) may need to focus on ridding their diet of inflammatory substances in order to boost their fertility. There's a lot of conflicting information on exactly which foods tend to be inflammatory. One reason for the controversy is in some people, foods can illicit an immune system response and inflammation, while other people have no reaction to those foods. The body can make antibodies to just about any food (and even your own tissue - which is the definition of autoimmune).

How do I know which foods have this impact on my body?

One method is to take blood tests that look for antibodies to different foods. Your health care provider should be able to requisition these tests. Another way to sleuth out counterproductive foods is by doing an elimination diet. You start by eliminating foods that commonly cause inflammation and then slowly add each food group back in while observing your reaction. For example, you may take wheat, dairy, soy and red meat out of your diet for three months. Other culprits include sugar, alcohol and coffee, though you should have already eliminated them if you are trying to conceive. Then, pick one of these food groups and add it back in. Eat it daily for a week and note your response. Do you have headaches? Digestive problems? Skin reactions? Fatigue? Inflammation? Pain? If so, take that food out and see if these symptoms decrease or disappear. If they do, then you know that this food group is not currently nourishing you. Once you have established your body's reaction to one food group, add in the next.

Thyroiditis

Graves' disease and Hashimoto Thyroiditis are two very common autoimmune syndromes that can lead to overactive and underactive thyroid glands. If you have hypothyroidism (underactive thyroid glands), you may need vitamin A palmate instead of betacarotene. Ask your health care provider which form of vitamin A is right for you.

Don't skimp on the whole grains. People with hypothyroidism need carbohydrates to support thyroid function. The Atkins (low-carbohydrate) diet, for example, wouldn't be indicated for those with hypothyroidism.

There is a whole world of vegetables from the sea. These veggies give your thyroid the key nutrient, iodine, needed to make thyroid hormones. There are several varieties of seaweed and many ways to incorporate them into tasty dishes. They are great in soups or mixed with rice, and make beans easier to digest.

On the other end of the spectrum, there are several foods that can suppress thyroid function called goitrogens. Peanuts, pine nuts, millet, soy and cruciferous vegetables (such as cauliflower, cabbage, bok choy, broccoli and similar green leaf vegetables) all fall into this category. The good news is that if you cook these foods, they loose their goitrogenic properties. So, simply cook your food! This is consistent with the OM dietary principals that you're already following, right?

Endometriosis

Let's tweak the East/West Fertility Diet just a little bit to serve your needs. Stay away from cheese and dairy. Season your diet with turmeric, ginger and flax seeds. Be sure to stay away from rancid oils. Refrigerate your olive oil. Keep your flax seed oil in the freezer. Avoid fried foods and don't eat roasted nuts. Love your liver by having at least one serving of sautéed or steamed greens per day. The cruciferous family of vegetables (such as cauliflower, cabbage, cress, bok choy, broccoli and similar green leaf vegetables) can help your liver process excess estrogen. Difficulty processing estrogen is common in endometriosis, so embrace this food group (just cook them first)! Keep your bowels moving, eat plenty of fiber and be sure you get enough water.

How much water is enough?

There are many different answers to that question. It depends on the context in which it's being asked. In the context of endometriosis, notice how much water you have to drink to keep your bowels moving. Sure, there will be a combination of factors, but given that you are eating plenty of fiber and vegetables, how much water do you need to be regular? Drink that much.

Detoxify Your Environment

We hear a lot about toxins in our environment in the news. What are these toxins and where are they? Unfortunately, these compounds are literally everywhere—in our water, fabric softeners, makeup, new mattresses, fertilizers, additives to our food, that new car smell… more places than you might expect. For the purposes of this book, we'll only focus on toxins that likely interfere with the endocrine system.

We're introduced to endocrine-disrupting chemicals (EDCs) in utero. Like all life on earth, we accumulate them over our lifetime. **According to researchers, exposure to EDCs "induces functional and behavioral abnormalities associated with reproduction."** Many EDCs target estrogen receptors on cells exerting estrogenic effects. These EDCs are called xenoestrogens. Both men and women have estrogen receptors on cells in their reproductive organs. They can affect male and female fertility, plus the reproductive and nervous system of the developing fetus. Xenoestrogens have an affinity for glands and tissues that regulate fertility such as the thyroid gland, ovaries and testes. Researchers have made connections between rising male and female infertility rates and exposure to xenoestrogens.

EDCs are a varied group, having different qualities. One of the ways EDCs exert such powerful effects is through biomagnification, a process defined by experts at Oxford University in 2008 as "…the sequence of processes in an ecosystem by which higher concentrations of a particular chemical, such as the pesticide DDT, are reached in organisms higher up the food chain generally through a series of prey-predator relationships." Due to their mercury content, there are warnings about eating excessive amounts of swordfish, shark and other fish that live longer and are at the top of the food chain. Mercury, a heavy metal, is an EDC that exemplifies this process. When we eat these fish, we absorb their mercury. Mercury can cross the placenta barrier and accumulate in fetal brain and kidney tissue. In addition to seafood, we can encounter mercury through vaccines, dental amalgams and skin creams. It's been linked to increased miscarriage rates and decreased progesterone levels. Cadmium, another heavy metal, can decrease follicle count, increase miscarriage rates and interfere with progesterone synthesis.

The conventional food industry uses fungicides, antibiotics and hormones in its products - which we ingest. Other environmental pollutants we encounter daily are: dioxins, lead, DDT and numerous other pesticides.

In animal studies, females exposed to bisphenol A (BPA) had a delayed and severely weakened LH surge. In addition to BPA, there is evidence that phthalates are common EDCs present in a variety of common products. Phthalates have been added to plastics to make them more pliable for almost 100 years. They're released into food and the air when a plastic container is heated. They're in the plastics we use to heat food in the microwave. They're also found in medical equipment, glues, and body care products.

Like phthalates, BPA is ubiquitous, also found in plastic as well as water supply pipes, canned foods and compact discs. Animal studies indicate that BPA exposure can affect the male offspring's sperm count for generations. Other hidden sources of these toxins are: toys, detergents and flame-retardants. As you can see, we're exposed to several EDCs through multiple sources every day.

Activities to Avoid

- Don't microwave food in plastic containers.
- Do not drink alcohol. Do not smoke. This goes for you too, guys.
- Don't eat sugar.
- Don't eat produce grown in countries where DDT and other pesticides, fertilizers and herbicides that are outlawed in the U.S. are freely used.
- Avoid/minimize exposure to electromagnetic fields (EMFs) found in cell phones, electric blankets and blue tooth devices.

Fertility Promoting Practices

- Check the recycle codes on the bottom of your plastic containers for a clue to BPA content. Plastics marked with recycle codes 3 or 7 may be made with BPA.
- Reduce your use of canned foods.
- Opt for glass, porcelain or stainless steel containers, particularly for hot food or liquids.
- Install high quality air filters (not just hepa filters) in your home and office.
- Educate yourself on the potential effects of arsenic poisoning (found in termite and other pest control formulas). One sign of arsenic toxicity is inflammatory conditions coupled with irregular hormone levels. For example, high levels of the hormone DHEA with low levels of other reproductive hormones.
- Chew your food. Remember that even though aflatoxins are natural, they are some of the most toxic substances on earth.
- Eat local and seasonal whole foods rather than processed foods. Find your local farmer's market. When buying produce, meats, and fish ask about the sources of your food and the conditions under which it was grown, harvested or raised.
- Switch from coffee to tea and avoid or at least cut down on the caffeine.
- Consider that tea and chocolate can counteract environmental toxicity. The polyphenol and antioxidant content of these foods makes them medicinal. The chocolate should be eaten in small quantities and only VERY dark chocolate with as little sugar as possible should be used.
- To counteract some of these toxins, include fruits such as avocados, carrots, beets, apples, oranges, purslane, kiwi, parsnips, dill, celery cilantro and parsley in your diet.
- To counteract the exposure to radiation that comes from air travel, take 2 tablespoons of olive oil the day before, day of and day after flying.
- Choose lean meats, even when the animals are organic and free range. Dioxins, a byproduct of the power industry, accumulate in the fat cells of mammals.
- Experiment with coconut oil, instead of butter, when cooking.
- Consider taking a prenatal vitamin rich in Vitamin E, A (from beta carotene) with Vitamin C and N-Acetyl Cysteine (NAC), selenium, folic acid and DHA. These all protect against the damage toxins can wreak on the reproductive system. NAC can counteract inadvertent exposure to DDT.
- Choose toilet paper and tampons made without bleach.
- Keep your immune system healthy. Regulation of the immune system is critically important for fertility. On the one hand, this means keeping viruses inactive. For example, the Human Papoloma Virus (HPV) can kill ovarian cells. On the other hand, if you are susceptible to autoimmune issues like Hashimoto's Thyroiditis, you may need to calm down some aspects of the immune system. Work with your holistic health care provider to keep your immune system in tip-top shape.
- Use water filters for drinking, and ideally, for showering as well.
- Do your best to identify the common sources of EDCs in your environment and minimize or eliminate them.

The American Society for Reproductive Medicine Takes on EDCs
In an article published in the journal, Fertility and Sterility, researchers summarized data on EDCs and their effects on female health. The results are staggering. They cited publications relating EDCs to ovarian disorders such as PCOS and irregular menses, uterine disorders such as endometriosis, fibroids and pregnancy loss, as well as breast problems such as breast cancer and reduced lactation. Researchers also discovered a link between the early onset of puberty and exposure to EDCs, and outlined the severity of potential negative effects of fetal and early life EDC exposure.

Stressing Out

We have discussed how daily stress is detrimental to fertility. It inhibits blood flow to the reproductive organs, disrupts hormone levels and increases oxidative damage.

OK, so, 1, 2, 3 stop stressing out. Did that work? Are you carefree now? If only it were that simple. We know stress isn't good for us. We know it's linked to several health conditions, including infertility. But how do we change our patterns? There are several options out there to help you de-stress. Keep looking until you find the right one for you.

For example, exercise can detoxify both body and mind. Get out and take a walk. Feel your breathing become a bit rapid and your heart rate increase as you pick up the pace to the point that you break a light sweat. Or perhaps try swimming, bike riding or yoga and see if these activities help you mellow out. Moderate exercise improves ovarian blood flow while heavy exercise can create oxidation and an acidic environment that can be counterproductive to fertility. So, don't overdo a good thing.

If you like yoga, I recommend a DVD made by my colleagues Brandon Horn and Wendy Yu, *Yoga for Ovarian Restoration* (available through amazon.com). Their program is comprised of different poses for each phase of your cycle to maximize blood flow and flush out toxins. Meditation, breathing exercises and vacation can all help you gain a healthy perspective on life, rather than feeling overwhelmed by the struggles of daily life and the flexibility. Sometimes I'll write "vacation" on a prescription pad and give it to patients to emphasize the importance of taking a break, even if that means just leaving town for the weekend. Lastly, be sure to get at least 7 hours of sleep per night. This simple practice will help you mentally and physically cope with the challenges of daily life.

For so many reasons, acupuncture treatment is critical for women looking to become pregnant, not the least of which is its capacity to reduce stress. There is an abundance of evidence showing the ability of acupuncture to exert calming and regulatory effects on the nervous system, provide blood flow to reproductive organs and help the endocrine system shift away from making the stress hormone cortisol in favor of making progesterone (the pro-gestation hormone).

There are so many improvements I need to make in my diet and in my life. How/where do I start?

Good question! The first step is always the hardest. I suggest that overwhelmed patients go slow. Don't change your diet for a week or two. However, when you go to the store or out to eat LOOK at what choices would be conducive to fertility. Stay off of the phone during lunch. Eat quietly, then use the rest of your time to go for a walk. Next to the white bread you typically grab, look for its whole grain alternative. Open your eyes to new possibilities by simply asking the question, "What else could I eat?" You'll be surprised by how many alternatives are out there.

When cooking, try different varieties of olive oil. Try a new fish recipe. Make *Meredith's Mini Muffins* and be amazed at how good they are. Wean yourself off sugar. Try xylitol or stevia instead of sugar in - what would be your regular cup of coffee - but is now tea.

Several small changes add up to big results. Realize that improving your lifestyle is a process, not an event. Lastly, take note of how you feel when you fall off the wagon. For example, if you've avoided sugar for two months, but then eat cake at a birthday party, ask yourself how you feel. You'll probably be surprised by the answer

Male Fertility Enhancement

IN 30-40% OF COUPLES with infertility worldwide, the "fault" of infertility lies with the male partner. In the United States alone, 3 million men have been diagnosed as infertile... and those are just the ones who are trying to have children! How many more men than this are incapable of fathering a child? Sperm counts have been declining over the past several decades. There are environmental reasons, and prenatal essence factors such maternal PCOS or paternal poor sperm quality. Are you surprised to learn that both of these prenatal factors can be detremental to a grown male's fertile potential? Postnatal influences include: immune disorders, environmental and dietary toxins, lifestyle habits and biological clocks (yes, men have them too!).

Much of male infertility remains unexplained. Yet, several known factors influence sperm count, health and function. Thus, there are ways to improve male fertility. I've seen men change their sperm motility (ability of the sperm to swim), morphology (sperm shape) and count through diet and lifestyle shifts, acupuncture treatment, herbal therapy and nutritional supplementation.

The Building Blocks of Fertility

Sperm are cells that are produced in the testicles. They are comprised of a head, which contains the father's genes and a tail that propels the sperm on its long journey towards an egg. According to the World Health Organization (WHO) a man who has at least 20 million sperm per one milliliter of semen is considered to have a normal sperm count. Only one out of the millions in a single semen ejaculate is needed to fertilize an egg.

This should be easy! What's the problem?

Here's the catch. Even though it takes only one sperm to penetrate an egg, the path to that egg is long and difficult. So, only a small number of sperm survive the journey. They have to be helped by cervical mucus, protected by seminal fluid and guided by the uterus and fallopian tubes. Not only are millions of sperm needed, they need to be well formed and able to swim forward quickly.

How do I know if I'm fertile?

That's a good question. There are many tests to assess male fertility: hormone levels, physical examination, semen analysis, the post-coital test, the "swim up" test and the egg penetration test. Physical examination and lab tests such as semen analysis and hormone levels can yield a lot of information about a man's virility.

Physical Examination

On physical examination, your physician looks for any physical or structural abnormalities that may contribute to infertility. One of the most common conditions that causes poor sperm counts revealed by a physical exam is a varicocele. A varicocele is a varicose vein in the testicular blood vessels. It causes swelling and irregular blood flow in the testicles, which leads to increased testicle temperature and/or hormonal imbalances. This blockage is a factor in up to 50% of infertile men, though it *is* possible to have a varicocele and have normal hormone levels and sperm analysis. The Western treatment for this is a procedure is called embolisation, which seals off the affected vein. While this surgery can be successful, it can also leave scar tissue and adhesions. Using OM in combination with Western treatment can minimize this fertility-reducing side effect.

Other markers assessed in a physical examination are penis and testicular size, hair recession patterns, muscle mass and breast size. Abnormal findings in any of these areas can give clues to the underlying cause of infertility. For example, small testicles could indicate an endocrine or congenital disorder. If hormone imbalances are suspected, your physician can order confirmatory saliva and/or a semen analysis.

The Semen Analysis

A semen analysis measures sperm count, morphology and motility. The quality of the seminal fluid is also determined, judged on its volume and viscosity. Today, a semen sample is considered normal if it is comprised of 1.5-5.0 ml of seminal fluid or ejaculate, with at least 20 million sperm per ml. While that sounds like a lot of sperm, the truth is that semen volume, sperm counts and quality have all decreased over the last 50 years. There must be enough seminal fluid to alter the acidic vaginal environment (cervical fluid helps too!) to a sperm-friendly alkaline environment. Healthy ejaculate behaves in a specific way after leaving the body. It first coagulates, then it liquefies. The number of white blood cells and anti-sperm antibodies in seminal fluid can affect its viscosity and give us clues as to what factors may be the source of poor sperm preformance.

WHO Standards for Measuring Male Fertility

Ideally, the sperm count should be well over 20 million; typically around 150 million. A count between 10 and 20 million is considered borderline density. Below 10 million is low and 5 million sperm or less per ejaculate is considered to be very low. Of these sperm, at least 75% should be alive, 14% should be well formed and 50% should show good progressive forward movement. The measurement of hyperactive sperm may also be included in a complete fertility semen analysis.

Interfering Factors

Sperm should not come into contact with a man's blood. If it does, the immune system can identify the sperm as foreign and produce antibodies to it. When antibodies invade the seminal fluid they attach themselves to sperm. This decreases motility and causes clumping (agglutination). This can dramatically reduce a man's fertility. Varicoceles, testicular trauma and injury, surgery (especially vasectomy repair) and prostate or testicular infections can also cause this condition. However, for many men with anti-sperm antibodies, there is no explainable cause.

If your semen analysis is normal, your physician may also order a DNA fragmentation test. Most scientists believe that DNA fragmentation levels are generally unrelated to other semen analysis markers. However, there is speculation that sperm with poor DNA intregrity may not swim very well. High levels of DNA fragmentation are implicated in infertility, failure of the embryo to develop, and an increased rate of miscarriage. The factors that affect DNA fragmentation also affect morphology and motility.

I have had 3 sperm analyses over the past year and they have all been normal. My highest sperm count was 88 million. However, my wife and I keep having miscarriages, for no apparent reason. It seems like she has had every test in the world, all of which are normal. Why hasn't my physician ordered a DNA fragmentation test?

In short, because there is nothing he or she can do to treat this condition. Unless there is an infection, blockage or a treatable hormonal issue, Western medicine doesn't have much to offer in terms of improving sperm counts and quality. Some reproductive endocrinologists in the San Francisco bay area are using nutritional supplementation to improve this semen paramater. Most Western physicians however, Rather, when faced with male infertility, most Western physicians only focus on filtering out the poorest quality sperm from the ejaculate before ART techniques such as IUI, IVF or ICSI (see the Assisted Reproductive Techniques chapter for more information). According to <u>Infertility in Practice</u>, a leading Western medicine reproductive endocrinology textbook, "The semen analysis has little or no relation to the underlying etiology and most treatments are based on enhancing sperm quality in vitro rather than treating the underlying dysfunction."

The good news is that you don't have to jump straight to ART. Once you understand the factors that may be contributing to your infertility, there are steps you can take to change your sperm quality!

Environmental Concerns

In 1940, the average sperm count of American men was 113 million sperm/ml. It declined sharply to 66 million by 1990. During this period seminal volume also decreased by 20%. Plus, the number of men with very low sperm counts had tripled.

These numbers indicate that the more recently a man is born, the lower his sperm count and seminal volume are likely to be. He also has a greater chance of having abnormally formed sperm. The dominant theory behind this dramatic shift in male potency is a complex interplay of environmental (possibly as far back as in the womb), dietary and lifestyle factors.

In OM, the quality and quantity of sperm is an expression of pre-heaven essence in men, analogous to egg supply in women. Sperm are yang in nature, as opposed to eggs, which are yin. While women are born with all of the eggs they will ever have, men produce sperm constantly. This is important. MEN PRODUCE SPERM CONSTANTLY. As a result, it is possible for a man to completely change his semen parameters within a 3-month period.

Men's potential for healthy sperm production depends on the development of their testicles in the womb. In fact, even prenatal exposure to chemicals can alter a man's potential to make healthy sperm. For example, the reproductive organs of males, whose mothers took certain drugs or were exposed to phthalates, (chemicals found in common items such as plastics, cosmetics, hairspray, shampoo and soap) were adversely affected, as was their fertility.

We live in a world rife with chemicals that can impact sperm production (spermatogenesis). While prenatal exposure to endocrine disrupting compounds (EDC) can alter a man's potency, so can postnatal exposure. Some of these chemicals act like estrogens (xenoestrogens), while others are directly anti-androgenic (they interfere with the action of testosterone). These substances are found in paints, polishes, plastic water bottles, degreasing agents, dyes and many other common items. Over a period of time, theses chemicals can build up in the body and hinder spermatogenesis. It follows that men wishing to improve their fertility should limit their exposure to pollutants, improve their diets and take antioxidants.

The Worldwide Trend in Male Infertility

Researchers in India found through animal studies that introduction to Bisphenol A (BPA), can significantly alter male's fertility. Humans come into regular contact with BPA through plastics. Male mice exposed to BPA fathered litters where there was a significant reduction in offspring, the male offspring had lower sperm counts and motility, and miscarriage rates were higher. This effect lasted for THREE GENERATIONS. At least THREE GENERATIONS of male mice (researchers only measured three generations) were altered by the effects of BPA on great-grand daddy mouse. While this is only an animal experiment (ethics prohibit this sort of experimentation on humans), the results are staggering.

But I don't handle toxins!

Did your great grandfather? Are you a mechanic, carpenter, painter, or avid home improvement weekend warrior? Do you drink bottled water? Minimize exposure by using gloves, masks and other protective gear, or simply avoid handling known toxins.

Simple Steps to Support Sperm Health

- Avoid bottled water in plastic containers
- Reheat foods and drink hot drinks in glass, ceramic or enamel containers - not plastic
- Wash all fruits and vegetables thoroughly to remove herbicide and pesticide residues
- Eat organic vegetables/animals and grass-fed meats whenever possible - especially beef and poultry as they may contain hormones and antibiotics
- Avoid eating fish species known to have high levels of mercury
- Buffer your exposure to chemicals with a diet rich in antioxidants. Good sources of antioxidants include vegetables and green or black tea.
- Soy contains plant-derived estrogens (phytoestrogens) so it should not be the main source of protein in a man's diet

Fertility Friendly Diet & Lifestyle

The East/West Fertility Diet is important for men to follow too! Men may need more animal protein rather than vegetable protein for optimal hormonal balance. It's crucial for both men and women to maintain a healthy body weight while trying to conceive. Just as obesity can impact the development of eggs in women, it can interfere with healthy sperm production in men.

In addition to a variety of health problems caused by obesity, overweight men tend to have lower sperm counts. Clinically obese men are 30% more likely to be subfertile and overweight men have a 20% chance of being infertile. Diabetes is a cause for poor fertility, in and of itself.

Diet and lifestyle improvements are easy to talk about, but for most people they are difficult to do. For example, the health benefits of quitting smoking and avoiding alcohol is common knowledge, but people still smoke and drink. In addition to all of the health risks ascribed to smoking, cigarettes also appear to decrease sperm numbers, motility and morphology. Nicotine seems to interfere with men's hypothalamic-pituitary axis, altering the levels of growth hormone and cortisol. Alcohol can have negative effects on sperm vitality and may increase miscarriage rates if consumed directly before conception. Marijuana can decrease the ability of sperm to penetrate the egg by altering sperm motility (early hyperactivation).

Specific Nutrients That May Bolster Male Fertility

- L-carnitine has been shown to increase both sperm count and motility
- Zinc levels tend to be lower in infertile men as this mineral is instrumental in sperm production, proper testosterone levels and sperm motility
- Vitamin B12, the subject of numerous male fertility studies, has been shown to increase sperm count and motility. In fact, one study showed that 27% of study participants with very low sperm count who increased their B12 intake had more than a five-fold increase in sperm numbers.
- Antioxidants help prevent sperm damage from free radicals. Vitamins C and E have demonstrated the ability to increase sperm count, motility and morphology. Additionally, in one study, vitamin E supplementation improved the ability of sperm to penetrate an egg.
- Essential Fatty Acids such as flax oil and fish oil can improve sperm cell energy production
- Folate is essential for safeguarding sperm DNA

For both men and women, OM theory asserts that fertility is the natural outcome of overall good health. Generally speaking, people are prescribed medications because there is a health issue that needs treatment. The disease being medicated, as well as the prescription drug itself, can influence fertility. Even common over-the-counter drugs like anti-histamines and anti-inflammatories (not to mention anti-depressants and Viagra) can be detrimental to semen health and sperm function.

Both men and women taking any prescription medications, should ask their health care provider how it could influence your fertility.

Mark's Story

I met Mark and Nancy when they made a Couple's Fertility appointment. As with most couples struggling to get pregnant, they both had health issues that impacted their fertility. Nancy had irregular cycles and hormonal imbalances. Mark suffered from erectile dysfunction (ED), frequent stomach pain and headaches. They had two children together and wanted a third. Nancy was in her late 20's while Mark was in his early 40's.

Both of them began and diligently followed the East/West Fertility Diet. They took herbal formulas, nutritional supplements and received regular acupuncture treatments. Over time, Nancy's cycles became regular, her BBT charts evolved to mimic textbook perfection. Her depression and constant muscle pain abated.

Mark had a different response. His pain disappeared rather quickly. However, after three months of treatment, he still struggled with ED, and casually mentioned one day that he had slight numbness in his feet and fatigue. Both Nancy and Mark decided not to have blood work or a semen analysis done at first. They wanted to wait to see if it was necessary. Given Mark's age, I felt he needed comprehensive blood work - at the very least. I suspected he was diabetic. He agreed to the blood work.

The results were staggering! Mark's cholesterol was sky high. But that wasn't the most worrisome result. His blood sugar was so high that I immediately suggested he go to the emergency room. He refused, saying that he didn't feel bad. He did agree, however, to retake the blood sugar test in addition to another blood test that indicates his average blood sugar over the previous three months.

He was diabetic. His blood sugar was again dangerously high and his average blood sugar result was high, even for a diabetic. I insisted he go see a Western physician and gave him several referrals to local Western physicians. Blood work in hand, he saw a physician's assistant and was diagnosed with high cholesterol and diabetes. He was prescribed two medications and told to report back in three months for repeat blood work.

Based on the Western diagnosis, I changed his treatment protocol to emphasize blood sugar support and focus on his ED. His ED had improved somewhat before he began taking his medications. But now something very odd was happening. During intercourse, he wasn't ejaculating. He could attain and maintain an erection (which he could not do before acupuncture treatment) but now "nothing came out". I suspected he was having a reaction to his medication called retrograde ejaculation. In retrograde ejaculation, the semen goes up into the bladder, instead of out the penis, during orgasm. I suggested he talk to his prescribing provider.

Mark was irate and wanted to stop all Western treatment. However, without it, his diabetes was out of control, not to mention his high cholesterol. To fulfill his fertility potential, he needed to become healthy enough to safely come off his medications. He also needed to change prescribing providers to one who was savvier about potential adverse fertility side effects.

Points to Ponder from Mark's Story

1. Fertility is an outgrowth of overall health. If you are having ED or infertility, it could be a sign of other health problems.
2. Integrative medicine may have saved his life. Had his diabetes and high cholesterol not been discovered and treated, chances are he would have died prematurely, not to mention that Mark and Nancy's chances of having another baby would have remained very low.
3. It is critically important to thoroughly research the medications you are taking to see if they could be contributing to infertility. It may be a rare side effect in one of the drugs you are prescribed. You can utilize your pharmacist as a resource to investigate any potential side effects.

Through utilizing Eastern and Western diagnosis and treatment, Mark's quality of life improved dramatically. His relationship with his wife is better, as both of their moods are more stable. He has more energy. He has remained free of headaches and stomachaches for months, and the feeling is returning to his toes. At the time of this writing, his story is still unfolding. He continues to make dramatic progress in becoming healthier - and of course more fertile.

In the pursuit of greater virility you just might find yourself leading a healthier, happier life!

Integrative Medicine & Male Fertility

Aside from lifestyle and dietary changes, international research shows that acupuncture and Chinese herbal formulas can have a positive impact on sperm count, morphology, motility and most importantly, pregnancy rates!

The subject of male infertility was not discussed extensively in classic Chinese medical texts. One reason for this was a cultural bias towards making women responsible for infertility. Also, they did not have microscopes to count and quantify sperm. However, as there is a complex history of treating gynecological health problems in OM, there is also long standing documentation of erectile dysfunction and low libido treatments.

Today, with our ability to see even the smallest of cells, we can measure the impact of OM treatment on specific aspects of fertility. There is a large and steadily growing body of literature supporting the age-old practice of improving male virility.

Potential Benefits of Acupuncture & Herbal Therapy for Men

- Resolve infertility related to anti-sperm antibodies produced by both men and women
- Improve sperm motility
- Increase seminal volume
- Increase blood circulation to the testicles and other male reproductive organs, including the treatment of varicoceles
- Improve overall sperm count and viability
- Enhance erectile function
- Protect testicle and sperm cells from the negative effects of dioxin
- Regulate testosterone levels

Well, if you believe in it, then it will work. I'm sure those men in the studies believed the treatments would work, so they did. But I don't believe in acupuncture or herbs.

I'm glad you brought up this point! Many people are convinced that OM therapies work through the placebo effect! Read the fascinating study from Germany below and perhaps you'll change your mind.

Correlation of Psychological Changes and Spermiogram (Semen Analysis) Improvements Following Acupuncture

Researchers wanted to know if semen analysis improvements were due to a "belief" that acupuncture treatment worked. Twenty-eight men were given both a psychological evaluation and a semen analysis. After acupuncture treatment, the same men took another semen analysis. There was a significant increase in sperm quality in all parameters but volume. The psychological test showed no change caused by acupuncture. To quote the authors, "Hence, we believe, that the effect of acupuncture on sperm quality is not caused by placebo-mechanisms."

But I thought you said that a semen analysis was not a completely accurate measurement of fertility?

Yes, you are right. A man could have several perfectly normal tests, but fail to impregnate his wife. Just as we discussed in previous chapters, his wife could score perfectly normal on every conceivable Western test and yet still not get pregnant. In this case, both men and women are diagnosed with idiopathic or unexplained infertility.

We know from ancient times that acupuncture and herbal formulas have been used to increase libido and virility. Now, with amazing advances in technology we can measure the effect of OM modalities on sperm quality and quantity. Ironically, while male infertility diagnosis has become more precise, Western treatments are lacking. We are learning that a perfect series of semen evaluations does not equal fertility. There is so much more to fertility than a score on a Western test. This is where OM excels. Practitioners look at a person's entire health profile. The nervous system, circulatory system, digestive system, etc. must all work optimally in addition to the reproductive system, for full fertility potential to be achieved. Thus, combining Western diagnostics with OM treatments opens up exciting new possibilities for improving men's fertility.

ART-East Meets West

THERE ARE SEVERAL TYPES of Western interventions in reproductive medicine. Hormonal medications, procedures that introduce semen directly into the uterus, surgery and in vitro fertilization (IVF) are all common Assisted Reproduction Techniques (ART). In the case of irregular ovulation, such as women with PCOS, hormones may be given to facilitate ovulation. If a woman is already ovulating, drugs may be prescribed to encourage the release of multiple eggs per month, thus increasing the odds of conception.

My patients represent a wide and varied range in experience with fertility enhancement. Each one has a unique path in their fertility journey. Some have just begun trying to conceive and want to start by focusing on improving their health. Others have been through several hormonal therapies, intra-uterine insemination (IUI) treatments or multiple IVF cycles. I've helped several patients go through Western treatment with donor sperm and donor eggs. In this chapter, we will discuss the mechanics of commonly employed ART and how OM can be used in conjunction with Western treatments to increase success rates.

Ovulation Promoting Drug Therapy

Women who are likely to consider ART as a first line option include those whose partners cannot produce sperm, those with blocked fallopian tubes, and women anxiously hearing their "biological clock tick"- such as those over the age of 38. This can be a stressful and confusing process for potential parents. International studies show that infertility and the progression to IVF can have a devastating impact on women's psychological health and marriage stability. Ironically, as we have discussed, the stress of an infertility diagnosis may cause the exact hormonal shifts that are implicated in unsuccessful IVF cycles.

After a year of trying with no success, my Dr. said it's time to consider ART and gave me a referral to a reproductive endocrinologist. I'm not sure. What are my options?

I hear this from many patients. An infertility diagnosis is given to couples who have been trying for one year, (if the woman is under 35) and six months if she is over 35. There are many different types of ART which a reproductive endocrinologist (RE) should be able to explain in detail. The most appropriate method for you depends on your age, your overall health, and the quality of the male partner's semen.

Physicians will often start otherwise healthy women under 38 with hormonal based therapies. These are geared towards promoting the ovulation of at least one, if not several, eggs per cycle. Two very common drugs prescribed for this purpose are clomiphene citrate (trade name Clomid) and letrozole (commonly known as Femara).

Clomid

Clomid is prescribed to stimulate the ovaries. It is commonly offered to women with irregular menses to induce ovulation. This drug has been in use since the 1960s, although exactly how it works is poorly understood. It appears to interfere with the hypothalamus-pituitary-ovarian axis feedback loop, decreasing the levels of some hormones while increasing others. While Clomid can cause ovulation in 70-85% of patients, it has several drawbacks. Because multiple eggs may be ovulated, Clomid carries an 11% increased chance of multiple births, it can also induce hormonal imbalances which can make conception more difficult.

Common side effects of Clomid include: hot flashes, night sweats, headaches, and vaginal dryness. In OM we view these as symptoms of yin and blood deficiency. One very important yin deficient effect that Clomid can cause is "hostile cervical mucus". This term describes cervical mucus that remains sticky and impenetrable during ovulation, rather than becoming stretchy. Hostile cervical mucus can prevent sperm from reaching the uterus, much less a waiting egg! There is also evidence that Clomid decreases blood flow to the uterus during the implantation and luteal phases of the menstrual cycle. This blood deficient side effect can make the uterine lining less hospitable to an arriving embryo. Small egg development, and inadequate production of progesterone are other potential consequences of Clomid use that decrease the likelihood of conception and increase the potential of early miscarriage.

Thus, it is common for an RE to combine Clomid with one or more IUIs during a treatment cycle. In order to increase the chances of conception, an IUI may be preformed on the day of or just before ovulation, as determined by LH surge predictor kits and ultrasounds. The process of IUI entails purifying the sperm sample and injecting it into the uterus. Just before an IUI, a semen sample is collected and "washed". Washing separates the poorly shaped, dead and slow moving sperm from the highly motile, well formed sperm. Ideally, the end product should contain 80-100% of the highest caliber sperm. In addition to decreasing the distance between start and finish, this process facilitates conception by guiding the sperm past the acidic vaginal environment, through the cervix. While this procedure bypasses the issue of hostile cervical fluid, if the endometrial lining is too thin, or the progesterone level too low, pregnancy may be unsuccessful, even if fertilization occurs.

Sounds like Clomid might help me ovulate, but can cause other problems that may interfere with my getting pregnant. Can acupuncture and herbs help offset these side effects?

Yes. Research has shown that acupuncture and Chinese herbal formulas can improve endometrial thickness. They also alleviate annoying side effects, such as headaches and night sweats. A study out of Sweden published in the *Journal of Human Reproduction* showed that electro-acupuncture can increase blood flow to the uterus, probably by regulating the nervous system. Investigators in China found that combining Clomid with Chinese herbs, safeguards cervical mucus and endometrial thickness. Patients in this trial took Chinese herbs with Clomid. They had almost double the pregnancy rate of the control group, who took Clomid with an estrogen supplement.

I tried Clomid and it didn't work. My doctor said I was "Clomid resistant". I'm not ready to jump into IVF, are there other hormone treatments that I could try first?

Clomid treatment is indicated for 3-6 cycles, as its peak efficacy is passed by cycle 3 or 4 and it stops working after 6 cycles. Femara may be prescribed as a Clomid alternative to women deemed "Clomid-resistant", meaning they don't ovulate with Clomid. It may also be prescribed to women who experience "Clomid failure", indicating they don't conceive even when ovulation is induced. Like Clomid, the goal of Femara therapy is to increase the number of eggs ovulated. *Unlike* Clomid, Femara has a shorter history of reproductive usage. Clomid has been used for about 50 years to induce ovulation, while Femara is relatively new to the scene. First formulated to treat breast cancer, it was discovered that the manner in which Femara impacts estrogen metabolism can be beneficial to anovulatory women. There is evidence that Femara can promote ovulation (couples still run the risk of multiples) without the fertility compromising side effects of poor endometrial lining development and hostile cervical fluid. Femara is slowly gaining popularity among physicians. However, there are conflicting studies regarding its safety. An IUI may still be done in conjunction with Femara, especially if the semen sample is of poor quality.

Gonadotropins

Gonadotropin drug therapy is another hormonal option, which is stronger than both Femara and Clomid. Gonadotropins (which include Gonal-F, Pergonal, Follistim, Repronex, among others) represent a wide range of ovulation-promoting drugs that work directly on the ovaries. Like Clomid and Femara, gonadotropins are given during the follicular phase of the cycle to stimulate egg growth. However, because they are so much stronger and carry greater risks, they are used for women who don't ovulate or those going through an IVF cycle. Protocols for administration and monitoring of gonadotropin therapy may differ between fertility clinics. Due to the strength of these drugs, the timing and dosing is carefully monitored so that each woman receives the right combination of gonadotropins at the right time in her cycle. Ideally, this therapy leads to ovulation, conception and pregnancy.

What's the downside?

As with all hormone-based fertility drugs, gonadotropin therapy can result in multiple pregnancies and increased risk of miscarriage. Additionally, the chances of developing Ovarian Hyperstimulation Syndrome (OHSS) are far greater with gonadotropin usage than with other types of ovulation induction. In OHSS too many follicles are activated, enlarging the ovaries and causing abdominal pain and distention. This complication can be life threatening and hospitalization may be necessary.

It Takes Two

I had an HSG and a saline ultrasound. My tests show no polyps or fibroids, my tubes are open and my hormones and glucose levels are normal. However, my husband's sperm count is low and the sperm he does have aren't shaped right and are too slow. What now?

Many people think of infertility as a woman's problem. As we have seen statistically, the cause of infertility lies with the male partner half of the time. Correcting a hormonal imbalance, treating an infection, giving anti-inflammatories (including steroids) or removing a varicocele, are common Western treatments for improving semen quality. Unlike OM, there are no Western medical therapies that improve sperm count, motility, and morphology in otherwise "healthy" men. Western options for infertile men often depend on the female's receptivity to treatments such as IUI or IVF. Hence, in this situation, while not infertile, the woman may have to undergo ART to fall pregnant. Women whose partners have particularly weak sperm may need to have IVF with intracytoplasmic sperm injection (ISCI). These therapies aim to make the most out of the sperm a man does produce.

Demystifying IVF

My husband's sperm count is 9 million. We tried Clomid with IUI and then Femara with IUI for several months. I ovulate and my lining is good, but my husband just doesn't seem to produce enough sperm. My doctor is encouraging us to do IVF. What should I do?

While protocols differ among fertility clinics, it is generally accepted that men need to have at least 12 million sperm for an IUI to be effective. Some clinics will discourage IUIs when there are less than 10 million sperm per sample. The basic principal is that the poorer the quality of semen, the higher the degree of Western intervention is necessary. IVF requires approximately 500,000 motile sperm. In cases where this many healthy sperm are not available, ICSI may be offered. This technique can make it possible for men with very low sperm counts or even no ejaculated sperm to become fathers. Sperm are collected either from the semen or gathered directly from the testicles. A single sperm is then inserted directly into a retrieved egg.

Improving ICSI with OM

ICSI works about 60% of the time. Researchers in China seeking to improve this statistic took a group of 164 men with very low sperm counts and divided them into two groups. The experimental group received herbal treatment for 2-3 months prior to ICSI. The control group only underwent ICSI. The density, motility and viability of sperm were all superior in the experimental group as compared to the control group. More importantly, fertilization and pregnancy rates were higher in the herb treatment group. Likewise, a different group of Chinese investigators demonstrated that OM treatment can increase the effectiveness of ICSI. They recruited men who had previously failed ICSI. After 8 weeks of acupuncture (only 60 days, not the 70-90 days required for full sperm development) ICSI was preformed again. Fertilization rates and embryo quality were significantly improved!

Wait, back up! What exactly is IVF? I read about it on the internet, but got confused trying to understand the process.

That's because it's confusing! In a nutshell, IVF consists of combining eggs and sperm outside of the woman's body, growing the embryos for 3-5 days, then placing them directly into the uterus where ideally, one will implant and pregnancy will be achieved. There are several drug regimens available to help accomplish this goal. The best course of action depends on the individual woman. The RE considers factors such as age, ovarian reserve and hormonal imbalances, before the correct plan is decided upon. In a natural cycle, typically one egg is ovulated. In an IVF cycle, upwards of 20+ eggs may be harvested. The ovarian response to drug protocols is carefully monitored through blood hormone tests and ultrasounds. The goal is to ripen as many eggs as possible without causing harm to the woman. When eggs reach maturity they are removed from the ovaries during a process called egg retrieval (ER).

At this point the eggs are introduced to sperm and fertilize. After a few days of incubation, the surviving embryos are evaluated and rated. Typically, the highest scoring embryo(s) are transferred into the uterus between the third and fifth days after fertilization. The timing of embryo transfer (ET) depends on the health of the embryos, the experience of the RE and the health of the woman. There are several risks to ovarian stimulation, some of which may cause cancellation of the cycle or freezing of all embryos until ET is safe.

To reduce the odds of multiple births, usually only one or two embryos are placed in the uterus at one time (unless the woman is over 35). After ET, it is up to the embryo to implant in a hopefully lush and inviting uterine lining. For the first two weeks following ET, many fertility clinics offer luteal phase support in the form of progesterone. It is discontinued if menstruation occurs or a pregnancy test comes back negative. Otherwise, many clinics suggest progesterone support through the first trimester. Embryos that were not transferred are frozen for future use, should the couple require them for additional IVF cycles. If pregnancy is not achieved, then some of the banked embryos are thawed and transferred during a future cycle. If pregnancy occurs followed by live birth, the couple may wait years before thawing out other embryos for transfer.

Those who have tried other methods of ART and not become pregnant are generally considered candidates for IVF. In women with blocked fallopian tubes or men with severe infertility, IVF may be their only chance for parenthood. Through IVF with a donor egg, even menopausal women, those with POF or ROS may achieve pregnancy. In this variation of IVF, eggs from a younger woman are fertilized and placed in the uterus. Donor sperm can also be used in IUI or IVF for lesbian women, single women, or women whose partners make very poor quality sperm.

Wow, IVF is expensive! Even without donor egg or ICSI, IVF costs thousands of dollars. What are the chances of success and I don't mean just a positive pregnancy test. I mean - what are my chances of delivering a healthy baby?

Good question! There are several factors predictive of IVF outcome. The most statistically significant one seems to be the age of the female partner. Almost 30% of women under 35 who undergo a single IVF cycle will carry a pregnancy to term, as compared to 10% of women between the ages of 40 and 42 and 1-3% of women aged 43-44. While not as dramatic, paternal age also impacts success rates. All aspects of sperm health deteriorate with age. Though IVF success rates are on the rise as the technology evolves, there is still plenty of room for improvement, as most couples do not conceive on the first IVF cycle. This has led researchers worldwide to examine the effects of acupuncture, electro-acupuncture, moxabustion and herbal medicinals in conjunction with ART and specifically IVF.

Several articles have been published since 2002 showing that women doing IVF who undergo specific acupuncture protocols before and after ET have a significantly higher rate of pregnancy and live birth. One meta-analysis (which is a review and statistical analysis of several research studies on a single subject) found that **acupuncture before and after ET can increase success rates by up to 65%.**

Over 800 Patients Strong

Over 10 years ago, a skeptical RE and an acupuncturist conducted a study in Colorado Springs. The RE didn't think acupuncture would help, but reasoned it couldn't hurt his patients. They developed a series of points, now deemed the Cridennda-Magarelli Acupuncture Protocol (CMAP) to give to patients during the IVF process. After a few years, they analyzed the data. The RE was shocked. Those who received 10 or more treatments prior to ET, and a treatment right after ET, experienced a 15% jump in live birth rates over those who didn't receive acupuncture. There were also fewer ectopic pregnancies and multiples in the acupuncture group. The most surprising aspect of the data came when they looked at which women got the most benefit. Older women and those whose partners had male factor infertility (poor sperm/semen quality) got the most out of treatment, with a 50% increase in live birth rates! With over 800 patients in their data pool, this is the largest study of an acupuncture protocol combined with IVF to date!

This research is very encouraging, but the clinical picture may be even better. Most research studies require that every patient receive the same acupuncture points and number of treatments. In practice, each patient is treated according to their individual diagnosis with a specific treatment plan that encompass acupuncture, herbal formulas and nutritional therapy. OM is based on empirical data, gathered from years of documentation of patient experiences. Thus, in keeping with the heart and soul of OM, it follows that this approach provides additional benefits.

East vs. West = Same Goal

Both OM and Western fertility enhancement protocols have the same goal – healthy babies. However, they approach this goal from very different perspectives. OM is holistic with minimal side effects and risks. It seeks to improve the prospective parent's health and thus their fertility. There are an infinite number of treatment options and herbal combinations that may be prescribed, depending on the nuances of an individual's diagnosis.

Western techniques are designed to over-stimulate the ovaries so that they produce more eggs, or facilitate conception by enabling weaker sperm to have a greater chance of fertilization. These ART practices increase the odds of conception, perhaps at the price of lowering the strength of the embryo. One approach is oriented towards quality and the other towards quantity. In OM terms we would say that Western treatments pull on the woman's pre-heaven essence, forcing her to produce more eggs. This approach may exact a toll, which can manifest as lower quality eggs, hostile cervical mucus, a thin endometrium, and potential health hazards. However, a big bonus to couples seeking to get pregnant is the speed at which ART can help them reach their goal. Where one round of Clomid with IUI may result in pregnancy, it may take three months or more of OM treatment to stabilize ovulation and change sperm motility and morphology.

OM and Western medicine have different strengths which can be combined to further their common goal - pregnancy!

Potential Benefits of an East-West Approach

- Increased ovarian response to hormone treatment — Some women don't ovulate even with heavy doses of hormones. OM can strengthen the ovaries, enabling them to ripen and release eggs.
- Fewer side effects of hormone treatment — Headaches, irritability and insomnia are just a few of the symptoms that OM can alleviate.
- Increased endometrium thickness — A good uterine lining is a well-known predictor of IVF success. If it is too thin, the odds of IVF failure or miscarriage increase.
- Increased implantation rates — After the embryo is transferred into the uterus, acupuncture and herbal formulas can be used to facilitate implantation.
- Improved semen quality — Western treatments can help infertile men become parents by reducing barriers to natural selection. IUIs make the sperm's swim shorter by placing it in the uterus. IVF takes the challenge of the journey away, while with ICSI, a sperm doesn't even have to penetrate the egg! Their offspring may pay a price. Male children are more likely to suffer from low testosterone, smaller testicle size, and poor semen quality. Thus, if a subfertile man could undergo three months of OM treatment to improve his semen quality prior to ART, he would be doing his sons a great favor.

Just as OM treatment can improve ART success rates, it can also undermine Western fertility treatments if used inappropriately. Great care must be exercised by the OM practitioner during ART, especially throughout an IVF cycle, to augment rather than counteract hormonal treatments. Additionally, unless a woman is a proven poor responder to ovulation induction treatments, herbal formulas that stimulate the ovaries should not be given in conjunction with drugs. Also, after the ovulation phase or ET, herbal formulas that invigorate the blood or acupuncture points that stimulate the uterus should only be employed by a highly trained fertility expert. For a list of practitioners certified in Oriental Reproductive Medicine visit the American Board of Oriental Reproductive Medicine's website: www.aborm.org.

Your Fertility Program

IN THIS CHAPTER WE will discuss clear steps to help you down your path of fertility enhancement. Keep in mind that there's no one universal plan of action. Some steps will interest you. Some steps you may have already taken. Other steps may not appeal or apply to you. Once you understand the principals behind fertility awareness enhancement and holistic treatment, you'll have tools to create a plan that fits your needs. This chapter's goal is to help you transform the information in this book into *Your Fertility Program*.

Keep Your Cool

Stress depletes prenatal and postnatal essence. It can decrease prenatal qi by causing the release of hormones, like cortisol, from the adrenals (the Chinese consider the adrenals as part of the Kidney organ system). It also interrupts the connection of the Bao Mai and Bao Luo. By damaging the organ systems essential for the production of postnatal essence, stress can lead to an insufficiency of blood and qi. Therefore, as you put your plan together, bear in mind that your first priority is reducing the stress in your life. Include activities that make you happy in Your Program. If you don't like doing yoga, don't do it! If taking your temperature every morning stresses you out, stop it! There are many paths to the same goal, taking the path of least stress is essential to success.

Acupuncture Reduces Infertility-Related Stress

Researchers in Sydney, Australia divided 32 women with infertility into two groups. One group received six sessions of acupuncture over two months while the other group received no treatment. Their findings are consistent with what I see in my clinic every day. The women in the acupuncture group felt less anxious overall, and had a significant reduction in relationship stress and perceived social pressure. They reported a sense of relaxation during treatment and an increased ability to cope with infertility challenges.

Don't Let the Stress of "Trying" Effect Your Relationship.

An important concept for couples is to remember that sexual activity is not just for reproduction. Sometimes when couples focus on fertility, they forget that intercourse should be a fun, nourishing act that brings them closer together. It can reduce stress and flood your system with opiates. There is evidence that regular sex may boost the immune system and regulate the menstrual cycle. Through opening the Bao Mai, loving intercourse can bring blood and essence to the uterus, strengthening your fertility.

Tips on How to Keep the Passion

- Don't let fertility become the sole focus of your relationship. Remember to keep doing what you love to do together such as bike riding, reading, hiking, etc. Spend time together where you DO NOT talk about fertility.
- Be spontaneous! There is only one week where you "have to" have sex for reproduction - the rest of the time is solely for pleasure.
- Also, don't forget the foreplay! Keeping this part of your sex life goes a long way towards keeping intercourse fun, intimate and enjoyable.
- Stress management is a key to fertility *and* a healthy, happy life. As you assemble Your Program, let this be your guiding principal.

Eat to Conceive in 14 Weeks

Regardless of your specific course of action for fertility, you will benefit from investing in your health. Make it a joint goal. In a heterosexual relationship, men should participate in these lifestyle changes EVEN IF their semen analysis is normal. In lesbian relationships, I encourage both women to take part in these life-encouraging practices, even if only one of them is undergoing fertility treatment. Single women undergoing fertility treatment should surround themselves with supportive friends and family members.

Begin with diet and exercise. Take an honest inventory of your diet and lifestyle. Are they conducive to fertility? If at first thought, your diet is "healthy", ask yourself how many cold, raw foods you eat on a daily basis. Could you substitute warm spinach salads for cold iceberg lettuce? Do you have protein with each meal? How often do you exercise? And perhaps most importantly, what improvements are you willing to make?

Making Improvements

Allowing a two-week grace period seems to astronomically increase chances of success. The first week, don't change a thing about your diet. Just notice what you eat, read labels - where is the hidden sugar? How many cups of coffee do you average per day? How long do you go without eating? The second week, set out to find alternatives. For example, if you want to cut out wheat, look for rice bread or crackers when you go shopping. There are even wheat and dairy free waffles available at health food stores. Take stock of your options. What you find might surprise you. What you thought would be an impossible task, may be easy. Frequent, protein rich snacks will cut your sugar cravings. Embracing the qualities of patience, resolve and consistency will carry you a long way in eating to conceive.

Lilly's Story

"I have a clean diet." and "I don't have that much sugar." Over my many years in practice, I've learned not to put much stock into these self-descriptive phrases. How people perceive the quality of their diet versus its fertility effectiveness can vary a great deal. Lilly's story exemplifies this difference.

Lilly was 42 when she made her first appointment with me. A self-composed, reserved woman, she was difficult to read. She described her fertility history and her desire to have a second child without emotion. She was overweight. From a fertility standpoint it would have behooved her to loose at least 15 lbs. She insisted that she had a "clean" diet. After her first visit, I laid out a treatment plan, which included abstaining from sugar. She listened, poker-faced and neither agreed nor disagreed.

The next time I saw her I asked how her dietary shifts where progressing. She said, "Fine." One look at her tongue and I knew nothing had changed. My other diagnostic techniques confirmed that her diet had not changed and she was not taking her herbal formula regularly.

At her third and last appointment, I asked about her sugar intake. She curtly replied "If my husband slaved for four hours on a desert, I am going to eat it." This was the first time I saw her express any emotion. Her response told me a lot. She was defensive, which demonstrated that she really didn't want to implement dietary change. Secondly, it indicated that these dietary changes were not supported at home. If avoiding sugar was the key to her fertility, her husband shouldn't be making desert at all.

I always encourage patients to be honest with me regarding the dietary shifts they are willing to make, as well as how many and what type of supplements they feel comfortable taking. It's best to spend your energy improving your diet, rather than wasting it avoiding difficult questions. You won't know what improvements you can achieve until you try. No one is perfect, just be honest with yourself and your health care practitioners.

Create Your Fertility Lifestyle

Read and make notes on the East/West Fertility Diet. Pay attention to the you can make to align your diet with your desire to conceive. If you have autoimmune issues, endometriosis, thyroiditis or other inflammatory conditions, consider cutting out wheat and dairy. While not everyone is "allergic" to these foods, dietary sensitivities to them are common. You can find wheat and dairy alternatives at your local health food store, and conventional markets as well.

Having Your Cake & Eating it Too

For most people, it's difficult to go without sugar. We crave sweets because our diets are filled with them. Honey, organic sugar, brown sugar and high fructose corn syrup are all high GI foods that are treated basically the same by the body. But, what if we could have our cake, and have it be good for us (or at least not as bad)? Polyols, (e.g. xylitol, sorbitol, mannitol, maltitol, mannitol) are commonly used as sugar replacements in "diabetic candy" and tooth-friendly gum. In addition to being low GI, they aid in colon health by drawing water to the stool and feeding gut-friendly bacteria rather than toxic organisms. A word to the wise: until you know how these polyols affect you, slowly introduce them into your diet. They are laxative in nature, eating too many may produce gas and possibly loose stools.

Get The RIGHT Amount Of Exercise

An international study found a correlation between increased levels of intense exercise and longer conception times in women of normal weight. Overweight women did not experience this impact. However, regardless of BMI, moderate exercise seemed to improve conception times. Fast cycling, aerobics, swimming, running, and gymnastics were considered vigorous, Brisk walking, golfing, gardening and brisk walking were classified as moderate activities. What can we learn from this study? No matter what your weight, moderate exercise should bolster fertility. Just as you can under-do exercise, you can overdo it as well. Women who weigh more are in less danger of "overdoing" it from a fertility perspective. So, choose your exercise program carefully, do an activity you enjoy, but don't overdo it.

Take Your Vitamins

Take a high-quality prenatal vitamin daily. There is evidence that taking additional folic acid or folate may decrease chances of birth defects. Common prenatal vitamins contain 800mcg of folic acid. Some women may choose to take an additional 800mcg for up to a year, or more, before conception. DHA is commonly suggested during the prenatal period. A component of fish oil, it has positive qualities for both mom and fetus. Some women notice something important when they first chart their cervical fluid changes during their cycle - they don't have any. In cases such as this, evening primrose oil taken during the follicular phase can facilitate fertile cervical fluid.

Spend your first two weeks setting the stage for improving your fertility. Get your diet in order. Decide on an exercise routine. Begin basic prenatal supplementation. Implement the entire FAM or pick aspects of it to incorporate into your life. Take this time to determine your ovulation detection/prediction method. Ideally, the male partner is open to taking a semen analysis. In the absence of obvious causes or blockages, a semen analysis can change dramatically in three months. Thus, he may be more motivated to adopt dietary and lifestyle improvements with you. Lastly, find an OM practitioner who specializes in fertility enhancement. The American Board of Oriental Reproductive Medicine maintains a current list of their members and how long they have been fellows of The Board at www.aborm.org.

Western Diagnostics & Treatment Options

Western fertility tests are incredibly useful. You may wish to begin your fertility journey with diagnostic tests, or wait for 6-12 months. If you haven't had a recent blood test and are over the age of 35, I suggest you get at least get a basic hormone panel. Tests can diagnose problems as well as monitor treatment progress. There are many tests available. I've categorized common fertility tests into the following three sections, based on a combination of expense and invasiveness.

1. Blood Work & Semen Analysis

This first category represents basic fertility measures. Men who have never fathered a child, have had a severe injury to the testicles, or work with chemicals should definitely have a preliminary semen analysis. Women over 35 who have attempted to conceive for six months or more, or those with irregular menses or unpredictable ovulation should begin with an annual exam and basic blood work. On the third day of menses, basic testing for women includes: estrodiol, progesterone, FSH, LH, prolactin, a complete metabolic panel, testosterone, vitamin D, and a thyroid panel. Any abnormalities should be followed up, either with additional blood work or imaging tests.

2. Follow Up Blood & Imaging Tests

If a semen analysis comes back as abnormal, men may want to seek OM treatment and repeat the test within one to twelve weeks. They might see a urologist for an exam. They may also get blood work including: testosterone, LH, FSH, a complete metabolic panel and sex-hormone binding globulin (SHBG).

Women with questionable blood test results may want to delve deeper by getting a SHBG and/or additional thyroid and metabolic testing. Those who receive an infertility diagnosis may follow up with a transvaginal ultrasound to check the ovaries, a saline ultrasound to check the uterus, and a hysterosalpingogram to check the fallopian tubes.

3. Procedures

At this point, men may follow a doctor's advice and do a testicular ultrasound and if varicoceles are found, possibly surgery to remove them. The equivalent for women may be a laporascopic procedure to remove endometriosis or uterine surgery to remove polyps or fibroids.

For more information on Western tests see the Appendix - Western Tests.

What Your Western Doctor May Say

Depending on your test results, your Western physician may offer women several options. Ovulation stimulating drugs may be offered with or without IUI for up to 6 cycles, though success rates decline after 3-4 cycles. Unless they seek out specialized training, most OB/GYN doctors usually do not offer infertility treatment beyond Clomid and possibly IUI. They often refer patients to reproductive endocrinologists for additional treatment and advanced testing.

There are some test results which clearly point to Western treatment. For example, blocked fallopian tubes, as shown by HSG, indicates IVF as the appropriate treatment. A PCOS patient is often prescribed metformin, and possibly Clomid if she does't start ovulating regularly.

Aside from diagnosis, duration of infertility also plays a part in deciding which therapies to employ. For example, if a couple has been trying to conceive for 10 years, and physicians are unable to determine the reason for their infertility, this couple may be directed strait to IVF. Other patients often encouraged to progress strait to IVF include women over 40, and couples where the man has a very low sperm count. IVF therapy is generally offered for a maximum of 6 cycles. For more information on Western infertility treatment options see the ART chapter.

Four Months Later & Beyond

By now you should have explored your options, made choices and plotted your fertility course. You have improved your diet and exercise routine. You know when you're ovulating and are making the most of that time. You've found an OM practitioner you work well with and you've decided on which Western testing, if any, best fits your needs.

I've done a lot of work! Now what?

First, be patient. This will keep your stress down. Enjoy the improved quality of life that is a benefit of a fertility friendly lifestyle.

Next, armed with the information in this book and a little self-awareness, you can make informed decisions as to where your path leads after 4 months. As a general guideline, if you're under 35 and have regular cycles, enjoy life and take further action after one year of trying. If you are over 35 and have been trying for more than six months, *plus* your cycles remain irregular, *and* you cannot tell if and when you are ovulating, travel down the road of ART. During these first 4 months of your journey, decide what additional steps you are willing to take.

Increase Your IVF Success Rates
1. Build Your Health Care Team

Your team should be comprised of people you connect with and trust. when choosing an RE, many women just look at the published success rates of each fertility clinic. This may not be the best approach. Some clinics refuse treatment to women with a low chance of conception, in order to keep their success rates high. Find out if this is the case. You should interview a perspective RE as if you are hiring them for a job – because you are. In addition to connecting with the RE, the clinic staff needs to be compassionate, responsive and punctual. You may already have an OB/GYN that you currently work with who can preform imaging and blood tests. If you like them, keep working with them.

Find an acupuncturist. First look at the American Board of Oriental Reproductive Medicine's practitioner listings at aborm.org. If there isn't anyone in your area, and your OG/GYN or RE can't recommend anyone, be ready to search online and make some calls. Before making your first appointment, ask questions such as: What is your experience with treating infertility? Have you treated infertility in conjunction with Western medicine? The answers to these questions will give you an idea of that acupuncturist's experience with fertility treatments. Do not ask if the practitioner treats infertility. You will almost always get a "yes" to this question as acupuncturists are trained as general practitioners able to treat a bit of everythi. the very least, get the "Paulus Protocol" acupuncture treatments before and transfer. Several studies show this protocol can produce dramatically increased ra of conception - up to two fold! A side effect of embryo transfer (ET) acupuncture treatments appears to be stress reduction. An American study demonstrated that women who received acupuncture pre and post ET scored much lower on stress inventory tests than women who did not. This study is another example of research that shows the effectiveness of acupuncture treatments to increase pregnancy rates.

2. IVF is Stressful! Have a Plan to Manage Your Stress

Find stress reduction techniques that work for you. While you won't be able to do vigorous exercise during the stimulation phase of IVF, ask your reproductive endocrinologist to recommend a moderate exercise program for you. Find a meditation or relaxation tape. Read mystery novels. In short, do whatever helps you relax throughout the entire IVF process.

3. Consider Herbal Formulas & Nutritional Supplements

I am a firm believer that herbal formulas should only be taken during an IVF cycle when prescribed by a qualified health care provider. Chinese herbs can increase the effects of ovulation inducing medications and prepare the endometrium for implantation. They must be prescribed carefully to maximize the positive benefits without increasing the risk of OHSS.

The information below is for educational purposes only. Your entire herb and supplement program, including your prenatal vitamins, dose of folic acid and DHA, should be custom-designed for you by a trained member of your health care team.

Hope for Poor Responders

A Japanese study published in the Journal of Pineal Research found that 3 milligrams of oral melatonin supplementation improved egg quality and pregnancy rates in a group of women who had previously failed IVF due to poor egg quality. It can affect levels of FSH and LH. Melatonin may also benefit women with endometriosis, PCOS and POF. Interestingly, there is also evidence that melatonin can help someone become pregnant, and aid the developing fetus as well. This powerful antioxidant can pass through the placenta and safeguard the fetus from oxidative damage. It may even reduce the chances of preeclampsia. More clinical trials are needed to fully understand the effects of melatonin in fertility and pregnancy.

Like melatonin, low levels of vitamin D3 have also been found in poor IVF responders. In fact, the amount of D3 in the ovaries is a predictor of IVF success! This vitamin is fat soluble, so it is possible to take too much. Ask your health care provider for a D3 blood test. The amount of D3 in the blood is correlates to the quantity of vitamin D3 in the ovaries. Your dose of D3 (if any) should be based on your laboratory result.

Lastly, L-arginine is an amino acid that may help poor IVF responders. There is evidence that L-arginine improves blood flow to the uterus and ovaries and enhances the effectiveness of ovulation promoting drugs. In addition to increasing ovarian responsiveness, researchers concluded that oral L-arginine supplementation may improve endometrial receptivity and pregnancy rates in poor IVF responders. Be cautious about taking L-arginine if you have genital herpes. This amino acid is hot in nature with an affinity for the reproductive organs. It can increase breakouts in people with genital herpes.

4. Clean Up Your Environment

Toxins such as Polychlorinated Biphenyls (PCBs) can still interfere with fertility during an IVF cycle. Researchers found that blood concentrations of PCBs at common levels in the U.S. population were associated with failed implantation in IVF cycles.

Guys, You're Also Part of the Program

In the Male Fertility Enhancement chapter, we discussed the effects of toxins and diet on all aspects of semen quality. Even though Western fertility treatment can make a sperm's job easier, the advances of ART may not be enough. Researchers found that men with idiopathic infertility or whose partners underwent an unsuccessful ART or IVF cycle had significantly higher levels of sperm DNA damage than their fertile counterparts.

It's important to avoid toxins and follow the East/West Fertility Diet. Even basic dietary shifts can improve sperm performance. For example, researchers found that saturated fat intake is associated with lower numbers of sperm, while consumption of omega 3 fats can improve sperm morphology. There is an abundance of evidence demonstrating that Chinese herbal formulas can improve seminal quality. Other herbs from around the world like Maca may also improve semen parameters. Take the nutritional supplements and herbal formulas prescribed to you by members of your health care team.

Remember, it's possible to drastically change your semen analysis results in just three months. Do you and your partner a favor. Even if your semen analysis is normal, participate in your partner's **Fertility Program**. Eat to father a child and see an OM practitioner at least once for a personalized herbal supplement treatment plan. If your semen analysis shows that you could use some help, utilize acupuncture therapy as well. After all, it does take two…

A Positive Pregnancy Test, Now What?

Be happy and cautious. There are many steps between a positive pregnancy test (also called a chemical pregnancy or CP) and a live birth. There are several conditions that influence miscarriage rates. Some we can control and others we cannot. Pregnancy loss increases with maternal and paternal age. It is also more common in ART and among people with autoimmune conditions. Many couples reduce their stress by waiting to share the news with friends and family until the first trimester is behind them. While this chapter is titled **Your Fertility Program**, it would be incomplete if I didn't touch upon the next stages after conception.

All pregnant women, should be hyper-vigilant in the preparation and selection of food

- Begin food preparation by washing your hands, food and all cooking utensils.
- Keep meats and fish separate from vegetables (i.e. don't cut up chicken, then slice carrots on the same cutting board without washing the cutting board in between).
- Don't let your food go bad! Cook vegetables and meats within two days of purchase.
- When in doubt, don't eat it. If something smells a little off, throw it out!

Pregnant women should avoid certain activities and foods

- Cleaning the cat litter box
- Standing for long periods of time
- Getting cold. Take a scarf and jacket with you at all times to protect your neck and belly from cold wind. Protect your reproductive organs from cold wind by wearing pants, unless you are in a warm environment.
- My first gynecology teacher used to say, "Don't shake the tree". Shaking the tree includes intercourse and nipple stimulation during the first trimester, vigorous physical exercise, and heavy lifting.
- Soft cheeses such as Brie
- Any potentially undercooked animal product such as: unpasteurized dairy, chicken, fish, meat, and eggs

- Any processed animal products such as hot dogs, deli meats and smoked fish

I highly suggest weekly acupuncture treatments for my female fertility patients through the first trimester. In my clinical experience, this drastically reduces miscarriages. If a patient has a history of miscarriage, or is spotting during pregnancy, I prescribe custom herbal formulas. There are several herbs in the Chinese herbal materia medica that can stabilize a pregnancy. This is another area where ancient wisdom is backed by modern research.

While this is an exciting time for newly pregnant women and their partners, often women don't feel great during the first twelve weeks of pregnancy. Fatigue, constipation, nausea, and food aversion are common difficulties of the first trimester. These conditions respond quite well to OM treatment. I find it beneficial to work closely with my patient's Western doctor to ensure the best possible early pregnancy care.

During the second and early third trimesters, pregnant patients most often come to me for pelvic or low back pain. It's common for pregnant women to use mild pain relievers. However, in both animal and human studies, use of analgesics are associated with fertility problems in the unborn child. Acupuncture is a time-honored and research supported method of pain relief in pregnancy. In fact, several studies find it more effective than physical therapy.

An article in the *Journal of the American Medical Association* demonstrated that a breach baby can be turned by stimulating a specific acupuncture point with moxabustion. Following that study, acupuncture techniques became known for this function in the West. This therapy is most successful if treatment is administered while the fetus still has room to comfortably turn, such as by week 33. OM medical therapies have been used to facilitate successful labor for centuries. Shortening the first phase of labor, ripening the cervix and reducing labor pain are all potential effects of acupuncture treatment.

In uneventful pregnancies (without urinary tract infections, pain, high blood pressure, skin issues, diabetes, breach position, etc.) I often won't see a patient again until the last month of her pregnancy. At this time, the "Pre-birth" acupuncture series is appropriate. These treatments are administered during the final four weeks of pregnancy to prepare women for labor. This protocol has been shown to reduce the overall time of labor and is also associated with fewer necessary medical interventions.

During the postpartum stage, mothers need to be kept warm. They have just lost a tremendous amount of qi and blood! Replenishing essence and encouraging lactation with herbs, soups, acupuncture, and moxabustion are common practices throughout China. The same gynecology teacher that warned against shaking the tree was also adamant that women shouldn't go on an outing with their babies for at least one month after labor. New mothers shouldn't immerse their hands in cold water by washing sheets during this time.

Common postpartum issues I treat include mastitis, insufficient lactation, pelvic pain and depression. I suggest preventative and proactive treatment for these issues. Get plenty of rest. Eat warm foods. Take herbal formulas and get prompt acupuncture treatment when needed.

Many Paths In the Fertility Journey

It might help you develop **Your Program** if you have some examples of successful approaches. As I've mentioned before, no two people are alike. Therefore, no two **Fertility Programs** will be identical. The following stories from my practice are presented to inspire you in your fertility journey.

All the Time in the World

In my New Patient Fertility Intake process, one of the questions asks how long you have been trying to conceive. Ellen was the first, and of this writing only, patient to write a date 8 months in the future! Not just a month or year, she wrote an exact date. I stared at the document for several minutes trying to process what I was reading as she began telling me her story. Ellen had never been pregnant, never tried to become pregnant, but she feared that she may not be able to. The date she wrote in her paperwork was her wedding date. While not quite 33, Ellen had concerns about her fertility because her cycle length was approximately 33 days and she had spotting. When she made her first appointment she did not know when or if she ovulated.

The prospect of having over half a year to work with someone on their fertility, before they started trying to conceive, was exciting. I had patients who wanted to construct their fertility strategy before a "problem" was diagnosed, but they had already been trying to conceive. I'd never had a patient who wanted to get ready to make the most out of her fertility almost a year in advance! Unlike most of my fertility patients, she had given herself the luxury of time. She knew she wanted to become pregnant, but did not have the stress so many patients have of wanting to get pregnant immediately.

We started slowly. First she shifted to the East/West Fertility Diet, forgoing alcohol and sugar. Her most recent blood work was done two years prior to our first visit. It showed an FSH/LH imbalance indicative of PCOS. Interestingly, the physician who ordered that blood work did not mention the hormonal irregularity to Ellen. I speculate this was because Ellen was thin and PCOS in thin women is seriously under diagnosed. She also had a menstrual spotting pattern associated with endometriosis.

Rather than test her hormone levels again, Ellen decided to put her resources into treatment. She started on folic acid, DHA and a comprehensive prenatal vitamin. Her weekly acupuncture treatment focused on pituitary regulation. She needed time to build her qi and blood through supplementing her postnatal essence.

Ellen's spotting ceased after four months of treatment. Through the FAM she learned that she consistently ovulated on day 18. She never needed to have blood work to reevaluate her hormone levels. She conceived the month she got married.

Twins Now

In sharp contrast to Ellen's story, Margaret came to me at age 41. She had been married to Mark for one year and they had attempted conception every month. When I asked Margaret what her ideal outcome would be, she was very clear. Without hesitation, she told me she wanted twins. Without missing a beat, I gave her the number of a good RE. OM, I explained, can increase the likelihood of conception of one child, but not multiples. I have never had a patient under my care spontaneously get pregnant with multiples. I believe that this is because OM's underlying strength is to promote the normal. One uterus, one child is the norm. Risks increase with multiples.

Knowing that her odds of having two children at her age was slim, Margaret decided to call the RE. We devised the most aggressive and accelerated Fertility Program possible. She underwent IVF and immediately became pregnant with twins. However, by week twelve one fetus had developed while the other had faded away. Margaret wanted twins, but was happy with one healthy baby. She delivered a bouncing baby boy at age 42.

Irregularly Regular

Alice came to me with severe endometriosis. She had suffered with disabling cramping during menses for 10 years. Though a young woman, Alice worried about her fertility. Her menstrual cycle was irregular. It varied between 21-72 days. If her cycle went beyond 28 days she suffered with PMDD, which manifested itself in emotional highs and lows. Mostly lows, she reported. She was clear that she was not trying to conceive now. Both her and her husband wanted to wait. However, she knew that endometriosis could be a deterrent to conception. In fact, she knew quite a bit about endometriosis, including the immune system malfunction associated with it and the increased risk of scar tissue near and in the reproductive organs.

The oral contraceptive pill, (OCP) is a common Western treatment for endometriosis. Alice had tried various OCPs with mixed results. In all, she felt like they contributed to headaches and increased her PMDD to such a degree that it outweighed any improvement in menstrual cramping. She wanted natural treatment for PMDD and endometriosis, as well as improvement in her overall health.

We worked together for several months. Her cycles averaged about 60 days, so three cycles equaled approximately six months. While her irregular menses was stubborn, the improvements she saw inspired her to keep trying. Almost immediately, her PMDD faded into a mild garden variety PMS which was "totally manageable". With each cycle the intensity of her menstrual cramping decreased until, after four cycles, it was dramatically reduced. The sixth cycle presented a challenge. Everything seemed to be going fine until about day 45. Then her body started giving her signals that she was going to start menstruating, except she never did. Her bowels slowed. Her emotions were erratic.

During this time she went out of town. So, she self-prescribed herbs, including a formula that I gave her with strict instructions to use only during menses to relieve cramping. Alice was accustomed to having irregular length cycles on a regular basis, but this was different. Desperate to bring on her period, she called me as soon as she was back in town. I agreed to fit her in during my lunch if she took a pregnancy test. Shocked at the concept that she could be pregnant, she agreed. Our meeting that day centered on her new pregnancy and planning for prenatal care.

Alice is a perfect example of a patient who fell pregnant, without trying, because her whole body became healthier. Her focus was not on conception, rather, it was on health and quality of life. Pregnancy was a happy side effect!

Moving Forward With Direction

Pattie was not a stranger to acupuncture and OM therapies. In fact, she'd been trying to conceive for 2 years. Now 29 years old, she and her husband decided to switch acupuncturists in favor of one who specialized in fertility enhancement.

She was very blunt with me on our first visit. She told me she had intermittently visited an acupuncturist, but acupuncture and fertility related therapies weren't covered by insurance and she had wanted to spend as little as possible. However, since that approach had not worked, she sought out a specialist in the field and was ready to commit to a fertility enhancement program. She wanted help through OM therapies *before starting down the road of ART. Her insurance did cover diagnostic tests. An overweight woman with irregular menses, her tests revealed the metabolic and hormonal markers for PCOS.*

She took the first three months to focus on furthering her fertility through dietary improvement, herbal formulas, nutritional supplements and acupuncture treatment. I utilized the Phasing Technique, changing acupuncture treatments and hormonal formulas to match each phase of her menstrual cycle. During ovulation, she received one acupuncture treatment and herbal formula. During menses, we used a completely different protocol. The changing modalities worked synergistically with each phase of her cycle to improve hormone balance, promote ovulation and increase her chances of conception. She was pregnant with a baby girl within five months.

½ Oriental Medicine + ½ Western Medicine = Baby

Jill combined equal amounts of Oriental and Western diagnostics and treatments. An acupuncturist herself, Jill was comfortable combining Oriental and Western medical approaches. She had every fertility related test imaginable, only to be diagnosed with unexplained infertility, which she found difficult to accept.

Her RE suggested first trying Clomid with IUI for four cycles before moving on to other hormonal treatments and/or IVF. Jill decided to do IUI, but rather than use drug therapy to ovulate, she opted to use OM techniques. Jill saw me regularly for three months prior to her first IUI. During this time I employed the Phasing Technique to strengthen each part of her menstrual cycle. She felt that her unexplained infertility was indicative of sub-optimal hormone function. So, she wanted to strengthen her body and promote normal hormonal fluctuations rather than override her body's natural rhythms with Clomid. Still, she did want to use an IUI to increase the chances of her husband's sperm making the long journey. His sperm count was within normal limits, but on the low side at 25 million sperm.

Jill was rewarded during the third IUI cycle with a positive pregnancy test.

Baby for OB/GYN

Holly was a sweet, kind person with big brown eyes. A practicing OB/GYN, I imagine that being in her care during labor is reassuring for many women. Unfortunately, Holly was diagnosed with unexplained infertility. Her husband had a poor semen analysis, and she had miscarried less than one year before our first visit. At age 36, Holly was hearing the clock tick. At her first appointment, she told me of her plan to do IVF. Her husband, a physician, would not adopt any nutritional changes or undergo any OM therapies to change his fertility. He felt that because they had *decided on IVF with ICSI, having a low sperm count with poor motility and morphology was "fine". This was many years ago, before data came out about sperm DNA being very important to the viability of an embryo. Seminal DNA is not necessarily correlated with semen analysis results.*

Interestingly, while he refused treatment, he fully supported her desire to undergo OM fertility therapies. Holly took herbal formulas and came in for regular acupuncture treatments. Her ovarian stimulation went very well. She produced more than 20 eggs! Of those, 16 fertilized and over 10 embryos made it to day three. They decided to transfer 2 embryos and freeze the rest. The result was a little boy I met 16 months later. Holly brought him in when he had a cough that just wouldn't go away. He was so beautiful - with Holly's big brown eyes.

One year later, Holly came in again. They had decided to have another baby and were going to do a frozen embryo transfer (FET). Again Holly became pregnant and after an uneventful pregnancy, gave birth to a little girl with big brown eyes.

More Joy for OB/GYNs

Shelly had watched Holly through her fertility journey. Both Shelly and her husband were OB/GYN doctors who worked in the same hospital as Holly. Shelly suffered from advanced endometriosis. The endometriosis was centered on her ovaries, completely covering one of them, and impairing the ability of the other one to respond to FSH.

Shelly came to me after her first failed IVF cycle. Her one functioning ovary barely responded to drug therapy, making a few small eggs. She had a story similar to Holly's in that her husband also scored poorly on all parameters of his semen analysis. The RE had not done ICSI, so none of those eggs had fertilized due to his poor quality sperm.

She approached her second IVF attempt very differently. First, she decided to switch to another fertility clinic. While farther away and more expensive, her new clinic's reputation exceeded her first choice. Second, she chose to work with Dr. Cliff, the same physician that helped Holly. Her first treatment was during the birth control phase of IVF. While a bit late to begin OM treatment, it was worth a try. She was uncomfortable using any OM modality other than acupuncture.

I saw Shelly twice before and twice during her stimulation phase. The fourth time she came in, she was in tears. She had just come from an ultrasound. Even though she was on the maximum allowable amount of ovulation stimulating drugs, her ovary was not responding. Dr. Cliff predicted she would have to cancel this cycle, but agreed to keep her on medication and recheck her in three days. I treated her with electro-acupuncture, using one of my strongest treatments to induce ovulation.

She came back three days later, after her next ultrasound. This time, her attitude was completely different. She had hope. There were now four eggs that would likely reach maturity. I treated her in the same manner, with instructions to come back right before ET. Dr. Cliff was amazed. He was able to extract five eggs and did ICSI on them all. They all fertilized.

I treated Shelly right before and immediately after ET with the Paulus Protocol. Two weeks later, she called to tell me she was pregnant. Nine months later she delivered a healthy baby boy.

Like Holly, Shelly made an appointment several years later. Now she and her family lived three hours away from me and two hours from Dr. Cliff. Still, rather than construct a new team closer to home, she decided to do a FET with us. She had three embryos left after the first IVF cycle. They all made it through the thawing process. I saw her just before and after ET. This time she gave birth to twins.

Holly and Shelly's babies helped comprise my first two baby boards (pictures of babies born with help from my clinic).

After Holly and Shelly's experience, Dr. Cliff became interested in OM. Years later, when I began my doctoral program, he served as my preceptor. We devised two research projects together, examining acupuncture's effects on IVF, and on Clomid therapy with IUI. One of these served as my doctoral thesis and propelled me deeper into my specialty of fertility enhancement.

Aging Gracefully - A Tale of Two Women

Agnes
Agnes had given birth when she was 21 and again at age 41. She wanted to have another baby and had no trouble getting pregnant. Staying pregnant was her challenge. After three miscarriages during the prior year, she had decided to come to me for help.

When I first saw her, I was struck by how profoundly her prenatal essence had been drained by her miscarriages. Her period remained irregular for the first three months of treatment. She struggled with night sweats and hot flashes.

Now at age 42, Agnes seemed to be going through hormonal changes consistent with perimenopause. Upon her request, I requisitioned blood work. FSH came back at

12.7. This level is higher than I like to see in my fertility patients, but not so high as to rule out the possibility of pregnancy. Rather than giving her clear answers, the hormone testing simply underscored the changing hormone levels that she was experiencing.

Thought it was very difficult, Agnes adhered to her **Fertility Program.** She was a daily alcohol drinker with a sweet tooth, so deciding to eat for fertility was a big change for her. After the third month, her menses came back. After the fourth month it became consistent. Slowly, her hot flashes diminished, as did her night sweats.

After six months of treatment, Agnes was pregnant again. This time, she was prepared. She dove right into taking an herbal formula time-tested to prevent miscarriage. She continued acupuncture weekly until she was through the first trimester - the time when she was most vulnerable to miscarriage. We worked with her nausea, constipation and fatigue. At eight weeks, Agnes heard her fetus' heart beat. Then, before she new it, she made it into the second trimester.

Agnes gave birth to a precious baby girl a few months later.

Jeanie
Jeanie was 40 when she made her first appointment. She was referred to me by a local acupuncturist who didn't specialize in fertility. It was obvious from the start that it was going to be difficult to help her conceive.

First of all, she had undergone nine abortions during her lifetime. Her most recent was less than five years before our first visit. Now, at the relatively young age of 40, Jeanie was experiencing perimenopausal symptoms. She had hot flashes and night sweats in addition to irregular menses that vacillated between 21 and 50 days. Her BBT chart displayed a sawtooth pattern. LH surge detectors didn't work for her, because she would have to use at least two per day for weeks on end. Even the OV-Watch was not reliable. It was challenging to determine if and when she ovulated.

After three cycles of treatment, Jeanie learned how to control her heat symptoms to a large degree. After following the East/West Fertility Diet, she recognized that she got hot flashes and night sweats with any sugar or alcohol. As long as she stayed away from these two substances, took her herbs with regularity, and received acupuncture treatment, she slept well.

I didn't know if she had finished with the reproductive phase of her life. I suspected this was the case, but couldn't be certain. No one knows when the spark of life will occur. So, her principal OM treatment had to support her process, whatever the outcome.

Jeanie tried to fall pregnant each cycle. She had timed intercourse whenever it looked like she may be fertile, as per her cervical fluid changes. In aiming to support her hormonal stability, longevity and health, my goal for Jeanie was graceful transition. While I didn't know what the future held for Jeanie, I knew her life was changing. Either she would be pregnant or cease menstruating within a couple of years. OM, in Jeanie's case, was applied to assist her in progressing smoothly into the next stages of her life.

As of this writing, Jeanie's story remains open ended. We all age, some of us more gracefully than others. The meridian system I chose as the cornerstone of her therapy guides people through life transitions. Either Jeanie is going to remain fertile for long enough to get pregnant again, or she is going to exit that stage of life and enter menopause. Either way, being free from hot flashes and night sweats will signify smooth sailing to where her body wants to be.

Family Building Through Adoption

There are several ways to create your family. Sometimes, after wrestling with infertility, people choose to live child free. Other times, they choose to adopt and/or foster children. Sometimes, even when one's **Fertility Program** *is solid, conception remains out of reach. It can be difficult for some people to come to terms with the insurmountable barriers to falling pregnant or carrying a child to term. The purpose of this book is empowerment through education, with the goal of increased fertility. Yet, I would be remiss not to address every fertility patient's worst fear: unremitting infertility.*

Jenny and Richard desperately wanted a baby. Both in their early thirties, they had been married for five years. During this time, Jenny had miscarried twice. She and Richard were clear on the parameters of their **Fertility Program** *. They decided to give pregnancy one more try, but if Jenny miscarried, they would not try again.*

They didn't want advanced genetic testing, or have a RE do a work-up. Both of them had health issues that impacted their fertility and quality of life, including dietary and lifestyle challenges, which they wanted to address with OM. They were not interested in ART.

After months of strong encouragement Jenny agreed to a thyroid test. The test revealed that she had Hashimoto's Thyroiditis. This put her at increased risk of recurrent miscarriage. She opted to visit a Naturopathic doctor for natural hormone replacement. We also worked with prenatal essence deficiency, which is how hypothyroidism is diagnosed in OM.

Richard's semen analysis showed a high level of white blood cells and a low sperm count. He also suffered for severe environmental and food allergies as well as food sensitivities. While he knew what substances elicited an allergic reaction, he didn't know what caused his severe stomach pain. His misguided immune system needed help. Cutting edge food sensitivity testing showed that Richard's immune system was aggravated by foods he ate every day. In OM terms we would say that the heat in his stomach, skin and intestines tainted and drained his prenatal essence, leaving him subfertile.

Jenny and Richard were patient. After following their **Fertility Program** *and seeing their health improve, it took a couple of months to gather the courage to try to conceive again. Within three months, Jenny was pregnant. She did not want to see an OB/GYN until the first trimester was nearly over. She set her first prenatal visit with a local OB/GYN for her thirteenth week.*

She cancelled that visit. While pregnant longer than she had ever been, Jenny miscarried in week 10. She and Richard were devastated. They were convinced that they would be "the best parents" and couldn't believe their God wanted them to go through life without children. They took some time to morn their loss. It truly was a loss for Jenny, as it seemed she would never have the opportunity to physically grow and nourish life. Richard grieved that he couldn't continue his ancestry. It appeared that their bloodlines would end with them.

When they were ready, Jenny and Richard started the adoption process. Through their grief, they kept the life sustaining habits learned through their **Fertility Program.** *A year later, they when they adopted a newborn son, they were healthy enough to stay up through the night and help each other raise their child and strengthen their family.*

Remember, It's *Your* Fertility Program

I've found that the majority of women who see me for fertility enhancement and are committed to creating and following their **Fertility Program** get pregnant and deliver healthy babies. The few who do not tell me that they rest in the fact that they did everything they could to have a baby. This knowledge gives them comfort as they transition to the next phase of their lives.

Each person's fertility journey is unique. Examining your options and developing an informed strategy that feels right for you is the key to success. It is my sincere wish that you use the information you learned from this book to create your best possible **Fertility Program.**

Notes

Chapter 1: The Roots of Fertility

1. Rapkin, A. and S. Winer, *Premenstrual Syndrome and Premenstrual Dysphoric Disorder: Quality of Life: Effective Treatments for PMS/PMDD.* Expert Rev Pharmacoeconomics Outcomes Res., 2009. **9**(2): p. 157-170.
2. Frackiewicz, E. and T. Shiovitz, *Evaluation and Management of Premenstrual Syndrome and Premenstrual Dysphoric Disorder.* J. Am Pharm Assoc, 2001. **41**(3).
3. Maciocia, G., *Obstretrics & Gynecology in Chinese Medicine.* 1998, New York: Churchill Livingstone.
4. Rochat De La Vallee, E., *The Essential Woman Female health and Fertility in Chinese Classical Texts.* 2007: Monkey Press
5. Wang, B., *Yellow Emperor's Canon of Internal Medicine.* 1997: China Science & Technology Press.

Chapter 2: Reading Your Body's Fertility Signals

1. Chen, B.Y., *Acupuncture normalizes dysfuction of hypothalmic-pituitary-ovarian axis.* Acupunct Electrother Res, 1997. 22(2):p. 97-108.
2. Ehling, D., *Enhance Fertility Using Chinese Herbal Medicine* 2009.
3. Ehling, D and K. Singer, *Gauging a woman's health by her fertility signals: integrating western with traditional chinese medical observations.* Altern Ther Health Med, 1999. 5(6): p. 70-83.
4. Lyttelton, J., *Treatment of Infertility with Chinese Medicine.* 2004, New York: Churchill Livingstone.

Chapter 3: Pregnancy and Fertility Challenges

1. Johnson, L. *Thyroid Disease.* in *Women's Herbal Symposium.* California, USA.
2. Poppe, K. and D. Glinoer, *Thyroid autoimmunity and hypothyroidism before and during pregnancy.* Hum Reprod Update, 2003. **9**(2): p. 149-61.
3. Chen, H.P., J.S. He, and G.S. Hu, *[Analysis on the traditional Chinese medicine syndromes of the patients with autoimmune thyroid diseases. Changes in the thyroid and immune functions in 109 cases].* Zhong Xi Yi Jie He Za Zhi, 1990. **10**(9): p. 538-9, 517.

4. Lima, A.P., M.D. Moura, and A.A.M. Rosa e Silva, *Prolactin and cortisol levels in women with endometriosis.* Brazilian Journal of Medical and Biological Research, 2006. **39**: p. 1121-1127.

5. Cheesman, K.L., et al., *Alterations in progesterone metabolism and luteal function in infertile women with endometriosis.* Fertil Steril, 1983. **40**(5): p. 590-5.

6. Szczepanska, M., et al., *Oxidative stress may be a piece in the endometriosis puzzle.* Fertil Steril, 2003. **79**(6): p. 1288-1293.

7. Hudson, T., *Women's Encyclopedia of Natural Medicine.* 1999, Los Angeles: Keats.

8. de Abreu, L.G., et al., *Laparoscopic Treatment of Endometriosis Focusing on Fertility Outcomes.* Expert Rev of Obstet Gynecol., 2008. **3**(2): p. 203-209.

9. Tanaka, T., et al., *A preliminary immunopharmacological study of an antiendometriotic herbal medicine, Keishi-bukuryo-gan.* Osaka City Med J, 1998. **44**(1): p. 117-24.

10. Wayne, P.M., et al., *Japanese-style acupuncture for endometriosis-related pelvic pain in adolescents and young women: results of a randomized sham-controlled trial.* J Pediatr Adolesc Gynecol, 2008. **21**(5): p. 247-57.

11. Wieser, F., et al., *Evolution of medical treatment for endometriosis: back to the roots?* Hum Reprod Update, 2007. **13**(5): p. 487-99.

12. Flower, A., et al., *Chinese herbal medicine for endometriosis.* Cochrane Database Syst Rev, 2009. **8**(3).

13. Wu, Y., L. Hua, and Y. Jin, *[Clinical study on endometrial ovarian cyst treated by integrated laparoscopy and Chinese herbal medicine].* Zhongguo Zhong Xi Yi Jie He Za Zhi, 2000. **20**(3): p. 183-6.

14. Stener-Victorin, E., E. Jedel, and L. Manneras, *Acupuncture in polycystic ovary syndrome: current experimental and clinical evidence.* J Neuroendocrinol, 2008. **20**(3): p. 290-8.

15. Tsilchorozidou, T., C. Overton, and G.S. Conway *The Pathophysiology of Polycystic Ovary Syndrome: Pathophysiology.* Medscape Ob/Gyn & Women's Health

16. Johnson, N.P., et al., *PCOSMIC: a multi-centre randomized trial in women with PolyCystic Ovary Syndrome evaluating Metformin for Infertility with Clomiphene.* Hum Reprod, 2010. **25**(7): p. 1675-83.

17. Xita, N. and A. Tsatsoulis, *Fetal Programming of Polycystic Ovary Syndrome by Androgen Excess: Evidence from Experimental, Clinical, and Genetic Association Studies.* J.Clin. Endocrinol. Metab. , 2006. **91**: p. 1660-1666.

18. Zhang, W.Y., G.Y. Huang, and J. Liu, *[Influences of acupuncture on infertility of rats with polycystic ovadian syndrome].* Zhongguo Zhong Xi Yi Jie He Za Zhi, 2009. **29**(11): p. 997-1000.

19. Balen, A., *Infertility in Practice.* 2008, London: Informa Healthcare.

20. Badawy, A. and A. Elnashar, *Treatment options for polycystic ovary syndrome.* Int J Womens Health, 2011. **3**: p. 25-35.

21. Lim, C.E. and W.S. Wong, *Current evidence of acupuncture on polycystic ovarian syndrome*. Gynecol Endocrinol, 2010. **26**(6): p. 473-8.

22. Stener-Victorin, E. and X. Wu, *Effects and mechanisms of acupuncture in the reproductive system*. Auton Neurosci, 2010. **157**(1-2): p. 46-51.

23. Johansson, J., et al., *Intense electroacupuncture normalizes insulin sensitivity, increases muscle GLUT4 content, and improves lipid profile in a rat model of polycystic ovary syndrome*. Am J Physiol Endocrinol Metab, 2010. **299**(4): p. E551-9.

24. Stener-Victorin, E., et al., *Effects of electro-acupuncture on anovulation in women with polycystic ovary syndrome*. Acta Obstet Gynecol Scand, 2000. **79**(3): p. 180-8.

25. Alieva, E.A., et al., *[The polycystic ovary syndrome and increased body mass]*. Acta Univ Palacki Olomuc Fac Med, 1990. **126**: p. 233-40.

26. Stener-Victorin, E., et al., *Steroid-induced polycystic ovaries in rats: effect of electro-acupuncture on concentrations of endothelin-1 and nerve growth factor (NGF), and expression of NGF mRNA in the ovaries, the adrenal glands, and the central nervous system*. Reprod Biol Endocrinol, 2003. **1**: p. 33.

27. Stener-Victorin, E., et al., *Low-frequency electroacupuncture and physical exercise decrease high muscle sympathetic nerve activity in polycystic ovary syndrome*. Am J Physiol Regul Integr Comp Physiol, 2009. **297**(2): p. R387-95.

28. Jedel, E., et al., *Impact of electroacupuncture and exercise on hyperandrogenism and oligo/amenorrhoea in women with polycystic ovary syndrome: A randomized controlled trial*. Am J Physiol Endocrinol Metab, 2010.

29. Cai, X., *Substitution of acupuncture for HCG in ovulation induction*. J Tradit Chin Med, 1997. **17**(2): p. 119-21.

30. Pak, S.C., et al., *Effect of Korean red ginseng extract in a steroid-induced polycystic ovary murine model*. Arch Pharm Res, 2009. **32**(3): p. 347-52.

31. Hou, J., J. Yu, and M. Wei, *Study on treatment of hyperandrogenism and hyperinsulinism in polycystic ovary syndrome with chinese herbal formula tian gui fang*. Zhonggou Zhong Xi Jie he Za Zhi, 2000. **20**(8): p. 589.

32. Ushiroyama, T., et al., *Effects of Unkej-to, an herbal medicine, on endocrine function and ovulation in women with high basal levels of lutenizing hormone secretion*. J. Reprod. Med. , 2001. **46**(5): p. 451-456.

33. Sakai, A., et al., *Induction of ovulation by Sairei-to for polycystic ovary syndrome patients*. Endocr. J., 1999. **46**(1): p. 217-220.

34. Shi, Y., et al., *[Observation on therapeutic effect of acupuncture combined with chinese herbs on polycystic ovary syndrome of kidney deficiency and phlegm stasis type]*. Zhongguo Zhen Jiu, 2009. **29**(2): p. 99-102.

35. Song, J.J., et al., *Progress of integrative Chinese and Western medicine in treating polycystic ovarian syndrome caused infertility*. Chin J Integr Med, 2006. **12**(4): p. 312-6.

36. Recabarren, S., et al., *Prenatal Testosterone Excess Reduces Sperm Count and Motility.* Endocrinology, 2008. **149**: p. 6444-6448.

37. Horn, B. and W. Yu, *Optimizing Ovarian Reserve.* 2010, Pro-D Seminars.

38. Krassas, G., P. Perros, and A. Kaprara, *Thyroid Autiommunity, Infertility and Miscarriage.* Expert Rev Endocrinol Metab., 2008. **3**(2): p. 127-136.

39. Trokoudes, K.M., N. Skordis, and M.K. Picolos, *Infertility and thyroid disorders.* Curr Opin Obstet Gynecol, 2006. **18**(4): p. 446-51.

40. Hu, G., et al., *A study on the clinical effect and immunological mechanism in the treatment of Hashimoto's thyroiditis by moxibustion.* J Tradit Chin Med, 1993. **13**(1): p. 14-8.

41. Kim, S.K. and H. Bae, *Acupuncture and immune modulation.* Auton Neurosci, 2010. **157**(1-2): p. 38-41.

42. Fu, B., X. Lun, and Y. Gong, *Effects of the combined therapy of acupuncture with herbal drugs on male immune infertility—a clinical report of 50 cases.* J Tradit Chin Med, 2005. **25**(3): p. 186-9.

43. *Measuring the Effectiveness of Chinese Herbal Medicine in Improving Female Fertility.*

44. Kovacs, P., et al., *TSH Level and Pregnancy Loss.* J Clin Endocrinol Metab, 2010. **95**(9): p. E44-48.

45. Lyttleton, J., *Treatment of Infertility with Chinese Medicine.* 2004, New York: Churchill Livingstone.

46. Li, T.C., et al., *Recurrent miscarriage: aetiology, management and prognosis.* Human Reproduction, 2002. **8**(No. 5): p. 463-481.

47. Zhang, H.Y., X.Z. Yu, and G.L. Wang, *[Preliminary report of the treatment of luteal phase defect by replenishing kidney. An analysis of 53 cases].* Zhongguo Zhong Xi Yi Jie He Za Zhi, 1992. **12**(8): p. 473-4, 452-3.

Chapter 4: Fertility Friendly Diet & Lifestyle

1. Boudarene, M., J.J. Legros, and M. Timsit-Berthier, *[Study of the stress response: role of anxiety, cortisol and DHEAs].* Encephale, 2002. **28**(2): p. 139-46.

2. Balk, J., et al., *The relationship between perceived stress, acupuncture, and pregnancy rates among IVF patients: a pilot study.* Complement Ther Clin Pract, 2010. **16**(3): p. 154-7.

3. Savbieasfahani, M., et al., *Developmental programming: differential effects of prenatal exposure to bisphenol-A or methoxychlor on reproductive function.* Endocrinology, 2006. **147**(12): p. 5956-66.

4. Crain, A.e.a., *Female reproductive disorders: the roles of endocrine- disrupting compounds and developmental timing.* Fertil Steril, 2008. **90**(4): p. 911-941.

5. Caserta, D., et al., *Environment and women's reproductive health.* human Reproduction Update, 2011. **0**(0): p. 1-16.

6. Salian, S., T. Doshi, and G. Vanage, *Perinatal exposure of rats to Bisphenol A affects the fertility of male offspring.* Life Sci, 2009. **85**(21-22): p. 742-52.

7. Meeker, J.D., et al., *Serum Concentrations of Polychlorinated Biphenyls (PCBs) in Relation to in Vitro Fertilization (IVF) Outcomes.* Environ Health Perspect, 2011.

8. Grasselli, F., et al., *Bisphenol A disrupts granulosa cell function.* Domest Anim Endocrinol, 2010. **39**(1): p. 34-9.

9. Cuspisti, S., et. al. , *Smoking is associated with increased free testosterone and fasting insulin levels in women with polycystic ovary syndrome, resulting in affravated insulin resistance.* Fertil Steril, 2010. **94**(2): p. 673-677.

10. Dunas, F. *Clinical and Historical Uses of Sexuality: An Oriental Medicine Perspective.* 2012. California: Lotus Institute of Integrative Medicine.

11. Pitchford, P., *Healing with Whole Foods Oriental Traditions and Modern Nutrition.* 1993, Berkeley: North Alantic Books.

12. Groll, J. and L. Groll, *Fertility Foods Optimize Ovulation and Conception Through Food Choices.* 2006, New York: Simon & Schuster.

13. Dunas, F. and P. Goldberg, *Passion Play.* 1997, New York: Penguin Putnam Inc.

14. Chavarro, J., W. Willette, and P. Skerrett, *The Fertility Diet.* 2008, New York: McGraw-Hill.

15. Bailey, C. and P. Giauque, *The Fertile Kitchen Cookbook Simple Recipes for Optimizing Your Fertility* 2009: 3L Publishing

16. Johansson, J., et al., *Intense electroacupuncture normalizes insulin sensitivity, increases muscle GLUT4 content, and improves lipid profile in a rat model of polycystic ovary syndrome.* Am J Physiol Endocrinol Metab, 2010. **299**(4): p. E551-9

17. Liang, F. and D. Koya, *Acupuncture: is it effective for treatment of insulin resistance?* Diabetes Obes Metab, 2010. **12**(7): p. 555-69.

18. Liu, Z.C., *[Effect of acupuncture and moxibustion on hypothalamus-pituitary-adrenal axis suffering from simple obesity].* Zhong Xi Yi Jie He Za Zhi, 1990. **10**(11): p. 656-9, 643-4.

19. Lustig, R., *The Truth About Sugar.* 2011, Santa Cruz Public Television: Santa Cruz.

20. Shamsi, M.B., et al., *DNA integrity and semen quality in men with low seminal antioxidant levels.* Mutat Res, 2009. **665**(1-2): p. 29-36

21. *Foods to Avoid During Pregnancy.* 2013; Available from: http://americanpregnancy.org/pregnancyhealth/foodstoavoid.html.

22. Stener-Victorin, E. and X. Wu, *Effects and mechanisms of acupuncture in the reproductive system.* Auton Neurosci, 2010. **157**(1-2): p. 46-51.

Chapter 5: Male Fertility Enhancement

1. Lyttleton, J., *Treatment of Infertility with Chinese Medicine.* 2004, New York: Churchill Livingstone.

2. Lewis, R., *The Infertility Cure*. 2004, New York: Hachette Book Group.

3. Chavarro, J., W. Willette, and P. Skerrett, *The Fertility Diet*. 2008, New York: McGraw-Hill.

4. Ramlau-Hansen, C.H., et al., *Parental infertility and semen quality in male offspring: a follow-up study*. Am J Epidemiol, 2007. **166**(5): p. 568-70.

5. Acharyya, S., S. Kanjilal, and A.K. Bhattacharyya, *Does human sperm nuclear DNA integrity affect embryo quality?* Indian J Exp Biol, 2005. **43**(11): p. 1016-22.

6. Fu, B., X. Lun, and Y. Gong, *Effects of the combined therapy of acupuncture with herbal drugs on male immune infertility—a clinical report of 50 cases*. J Tradit Chin Med, 2005. **25**(3): p. 186-9.

7. Jeng, H., et al., *A substance isolated from Cornus officinalis enhances the motility of human sperm*. Am J Chin Med, 1997. **25**: p. 301-306.

8. Attaman, J.A.e.a., *Dietary fat and semen quality among men attending a fertility clinic*. Human Reproduction, 2012. **0**(0): p. 1-9.

9. Recabarren, S., et al., *Prenatal Testosterone Excess Reduces Sperm Count and Motility*. Endocrinology, 2008. **149**: p. 6444-6448.

10. Recabarren, S., et al., *Metabolic Profile in Sons of Women with Polycystic Ovary Syndrome*. Journal of Clinical Endocrinology & Metabolism, 2008. **93**(5): p. 1820-1826.

11. Sinclair, S., *Male infertility: nutritional and environmental considerations*. Altern Med Rev, 2000. **5**(1): p. 28-38.

12. Boxmeer, J., M. Smit, and E. Utomo, *Low folate in seminal plasma is associated with increased sperm DNA damage*. Fertil Steril, 2009. **92**: p. 548-556.

13. Sun, J. and A.F. Zhou, *[Damage to and protection of sperm DNA]*. Zhonghua Nan Ke Xue, 2006. **12**(7): p. 639-42, 646.

14. Shamsi, M.B., et al., *DNA integrity and semen quality in men with low seminal antioxidant levels*. Mutat Res, 2009. **665**(1-2): p. 29-36.

15. Meeker, J.D., et al., *Urinary concentrations of parabens and serum hormone levels, semen quality parameters, and sperm DNA damage*. Environ Health Perspect, 2011. **119**(2): p. 252-7.

16. Hofny, E., et al., *Semen parameters and hormonal profile in obese fertile and infertile males*. Fertil Steril, 2010. **94**(2): p. 581-584.

17. Fisch, H., *Older men are having children, but the reality of a male biological clock makes this trend worrisome*. Geriatrics, 2009. **64**(1): p. 14-7.

18. Pei, J., et al., *Quantitative evaluation of spermatozoa ultrastructure after acupuncture treatment for idiopathic male infertility*. Fertil Steril, 2005. **84**: p. 141-147.

19. Cakmak, Y., et al., *Point- and frequency-specific response of the testicular artery to abdominal electroacupuncture in humans*. Fertil Steril, 2008. **90**: p. 1732-1738.

20. Siterman, S., et al., *Effect of acupuncture on sperm parameters of males suffering from subfertility related to low sperm quality*. Arch Androl, 1997. **39**(2): p. 155-161.

21. Riegler, R., et al., *[Correlation of psychological changes and spermiogram improvements following acupuncture].* Urologe A, 1984. **23**(6): p. 329-33.
22. Kim, S.K. and H. Bae, *Acupuncture and immune modulation.* Auton Neurosci, 2010. **157**(1-2): p. 38-41.
23. Ishikawa, H., et al., *Effects of guizhi-fuling-wan on male infertility with varicocele.* Am J Chin Med, 1996. **24**: p. 327-331.
24. Fischl, F., et al., *[Modification of semen quality by acupuncture in subfertile males].* Geburtshilfe Frauenheilkd, 1984. **44**(8): p. 510-2.
25. Dieterle, S., et al., *A prospective randomized placebo-controlled study of the effect of acupuncture in infertile patients with severe oligoasthenozoospermia.* Fertil Steril, 2009. **92**(4): p. 1340-3.
26. Deadman, P., *Male Infertility.* 2010, Pro-D Seminars.
27. Balen, A., *Infertility in Practice.* 2008, London: Informa Healthcare.
28. Domar, A., et. al, *The risks of selective serotonin reuptake inhibitor use in infertile women: a review of the impact on fertility, pregnancy, neonatal health and beyond.* Human Reproduction, 2012. **0**: p. 1-12.
29. Gonzales, G.e.a., *Lepidium meyenli (Maca): A Plant from the Highlands of Peru-from Tradition to Science.* Research in Complementary Medicine, 2009. **16**(6).

Chapter 6: Assisted Reproductive Techniques: East Meets West

1. Smeenk, J.M.J., et al., *Stress and outcome success in IVF: the role of self-reports and endocrine variables.* Human Reproduction, 2004. **20**(4): p. 991-996.
2. Dieterle, S., et al., *A prospective randomized placebo-controlled study of the effect of acupuncture in infertile patients with severe oligoasthenozoospermia.* Fertil Steril, 2009. **92**(4): p. 1340-3.
3. Cui, W., et al., *[Effects of electroacupuncture on in vitro fertilization and embryo transplantation in the patient of infertility with different syndromes].* Zhongguo Zhen Jiu, 2008. **28**(4): p. 254-6.
4. Chen, J., et al., *[Effects of electroacupuncture on in vitro fertilization-embryo transfer (IVF-ET) of patients with poor ovarian response].* Zhongguo Zhen Jiu, 2009. **29**(10): p. 775-9.
5. Bukulmez, O., *Does assisted reproductive technology cause birth defects?* Curr Opin Obstet Gynecol, 2009. **21**(3): p. 260-4.
6. Benson, M.R., et al., *IMPACT OF ACUPUNCTURE BEFORE AND AFTER EMBRYO TRANSFER ON THE OUTCOME OF IN VITRO FERTILIZATION CYCLES: A PROSPECTIVE SINGLE BLIND RANDOMIZED STUDY.* Fertil Steril. **Supplement**: p. 35.
7. *Acupuncture and Chinese herbal treatment for women undergoing intrauterine insemination.* Eur J Integr Med, 2011.
8. Rozenn, M., *Acupuncture with Clomid and Intrauterine Insemination for Unexplained Infertility.* 2009.

9. Hsu, C., Kuo, HC, Wang, ST., Huang, KE., *Interference with uterine blood flow by clomiphene citrate in women with unexplained infertility.* Obstert Gynecol. , 1995. **86**(6): p. 917-921.

10. Wang, X., et al., *Vitamin C and Vitamin E supplementation reduce oxidative stress–induced embryo toxicity and improve the blastocyst development rate.* 78, 2002. **6**: p. 1272-1277.

11. Ozkan, S., et al., *Replete vitamin D stores predict reproductive success following in vitro fertilization.* Fertil Steril, 2010. **94**: p. 1314-1319.

12. Tang, T., et al., *Insulin-sensitising drugs (metformin, rosiglitazone, pioglitazone, D-chiro-inositol) for women with polycystic ovary syndrome, oligo amenorrhoea and subfertility.* Cochrane Database Syst Rev, 2010(1): p. CD003053.

13. Lian, F., Y. Teng, and J. Zhang, *Clinical study on effect of Erzhi Tiangui Granule in improving the quality of oocytes and leukemia inhibitory factor in follicular fluid of women undergoing in vitro fertilization and embryo transfer.* Zhongguo Zhong Xi Yi Jie He Za Zhi, 2007. **27**(11): p. 976-979.

14. Lian, F., Z. Sun, and J. Zhang, *Combined therapy of Chinese medicine with in vitro fertilization and embryo transplantation for treatment of polycystic ovarian syndrome.* Zhongguo Zhong Xi Yi Jie He Za Zhi, 2008. **11**: p. 977-980.

15. Lian, F., et al., *Effect of Quyu Jiedu Granule () on microenvironment of ova in patients with endometriosis.* Chin J Integr Med, 2009. **1**: p. 42-46.

16. Battaglia, C., et al., *Adjuvant L-arginine treatment for in-vitro fertilization in poor responder patients.* Human Reproduction, 1999. **14**(7): p. 1690-1697.

17. Ramlau-Hansen, C.H., et al., *Parental infertility and semen quality in male off-spring: a follow-up study.* Am J Epidemiol, 2007. **166**(5): p. 568-70.

18. Mau Kai, C., et al., *Reduced serum testosterone levels in infant boys conceived by intracytoplasmic sperm injection.* J Clin Endocrinol Metab, 2007. **92**(7): p. 2598-603.

19. Jensen, T.K., et al., *Fertility treatment and reproductive health of male offspring: a study of 1,925 young men from the general population.* Am J Epidemiol, 2007. **165**(5): p. 583-90.

20. Alukal, J.P. and D.J. Lamb, *Intracytoplasmic sperm injection (ICSI)—what are the risks?* Urol Clin North Am, 2008. **35**(2): p. 277-88, ix-x.

21. Shao, F.M., X.B. Zhu, and Z. Li, *[Genetic risks of intracytoplasmic sperm injection for male infertility].* Zhonghua Nan Ke Xue, 2008. **14**(1): p. 71-4.

22. Lian, F., N. Zhang, and J.W. Zhang, *[Clinical observation on effect of zhenqi zhuanyin decoction combined with intrauterine insemination in treating spleen-kidney deficiency type patients of sterility with positive anti-sperm antibody].* Zhongguo Zhong Xi Yi Jie He Za Zhi, 2002. **22**(2): p. 95-7.

23. Avendano, C., et al., *DNA fragmentation of normal spermatozoa negatively impacts embryo quality and intracytoplasmic sperm injection outcome.* Fertil Steril, 2010. **94**(2): p. 549-57.

24. Acharyya, S., S. Kanjilal, and A.K. Bhattacharyya, *Does human sperm nuclear DNA integrity affect embryo quality?* Indian J Exp Biol, 2005. **43**(11): p. 1016-22.

25. Meeker, J.D., et al., *Serum Concentrations of Polychlorinated Biphenyls (PCBs) in Relation to in Vitro Fertilization (IVF) Outcomes.* Environ Health Perspect, 2011.

26. Meeker, J.D., et al., *Urinary concentrations of parabens and serum hormone levels, semen quality parameters, and sperm DNA damage.* Environ Health Perspect, 2011. **119**(2): p. 252-7.

27. Simona, J., et al., *Effect of polychlorinated biphenyls (PCBs) and 1,1,1-tri-chloro-2,2,-bis (4-chlorophenyl)-ethane (DDT) in follicular fluid on the results of in vitro fertilization–embryo transfer (IVF-ET) programs.* Fertil Steril, 2010. **93**: p. 1831-1836.

28. Coyle, C. and C. Smith, *A survey comparing TCM diagnosis, health status and medical diagnosis in women undergoing assisted reproduction.* Acupuncture in Medicine, 2005. **23**(2): p. 62-69.

29. De Lacey, S., C.A. Smith, and C. Paterson, *Building resilience: a preliminary exploration of women's perceptions of the use of acupuncture as an adjunct to In Vitro Fertilisation.* BMC Complement Altern Med, 2009. **9**: p. 50.

30. Lok, I.H., et al., *Psychiatric morbidity amongst infertile Chinese women undergoing treatment with assisted reproductive technology and the impact of treatment failure.* Gynecol Obstet Invest, 2002. **53**(4): p. 195-9.

31. Csemiczky, G., B.M. Landgren, and A. Collins, *The influence of stress and state anxiety on the outcome of IVF-treatment: psychological and endocrinological assessment of Swedish women entering IVF-treatment.* Acta Obstet Gynecol Scand, 2000. **79**(2): p. 113-8.

32. Balk, J., et al., *The relationship between perceived stress, acupuncture, and pregnancy rates among IVF patients: a pilot study.* Complement Ther Clin Pract, 2010. **16**(3): p. 154-7.

33. Adams, M.L., et al., *The role of endogenous peptides in the action of opioid analgesics.* Ann Emerg Med, 1986. **15**(9): p. 1030-5.

34. Avendano, C., et al., *DNA fragmentation of normal spermatozoa negatively impacts embryo quality and intracytoplasmic sperm injection outcome.* Fertil Steril, 2010. **94**(2).

35. Lyttleton, J., *Treatment of Infertility with Chinese Medicine.* 2004, New York: Churchill Livingstone.

36. Liang, L., *Acupuncture & IVF Increaase IVF Success by 40-60%.* 2003, Boulder: Blue Poppy.

37. Lewis, R., *The Infertility Cure.* 2004, New York: Hachette Book Group.

38. Cridennda, D.K., *Summary of Acupuncture Studies related to Reproductive Medicine* 2012.

39. Rubio, R., *A Comprehensive Review of Studies Related to Chinese Herbal Medicine and Traditional Chinese Medicine (TCM) in Conjunction with Assisted ReproductiveTechnology (ART), IVF, and IUI for Male and Female Infertility.*

40. Song, F.J., S.L. Zheng, and D.Z. Ma, *[Clinical observation on acupuncture for treatment of infertility of ovulatory disturbance].* Zhongguo Zhen Jiu, 2008. **28**(1): p. 21-3.

41. Singh, S., *Ovulation Induction, Overview of Medications and Their TCM Translation.* 2010, Yo San University.

42. Fisch, H., *Older men are having children, but the reality of a male biological clock makes this trend worrisome.* Geriatrics, 2009. **64**(1): p. 14-7.

43. Hellmann, O. and Y. Bentov, *[Congenital malformations in children born after IVF].* Harefuah, 2005. **144**(12): p. 852-8, 910.

Chapter 7: Your Fertility Program

1. Rubio, R., *A Comprehensive Review of Studies Related to Chinese Herbal Medicine and Traditional Chinese Medicine (TCM) in Conjunction with Assisted ReproductiveTechnology (ART), IVF, and IUI for Male and Female Infertility.*

2. Ozkan, S., et al., *Replete vitamin D stores predict reproductive success following in vitro fertilization.* Fertil Steril, 2010. **94**: p. 1314-1319.

3. Cridennda, D.K., *Summary of Acupuncture Studies related to Reproductive Medicine* 2012.

4. Reiter, R.e.a., *Melatonin and Reproduction Revisited.* Biol Reprod, 2009. **81**(3 445-456).

5. Lian, F., Y. Teng, and J. Zhang, *Clinical study on effect of Erzhi Tiangui Granule in improving the quality of oocytes and leukemia inhibitory factor in follicular fluid of women undergoing in vitro fertilization and embryo transfer.* Zhongguo Zhong Xi Yi Jie He Za Zhi, 2007. **27**(11): p. 976-979.

6. Curtis, P., R. Coeytaux, and P. Hapke, *Acupuncture for Birth Preparation and Delivery: How Investigating Mechanisms of Action Can Generate Research.* Complementary Health Practice Review, 2006. **11**(176).

7. Chen, J. and T. Chen, *Chinese Medical Herbology and Pharmacology.* 2001, City of Industry: Art of Medicine Press.

8. Lyttleton, J., *Treatment of Infertility with Chinese Medicine.* 2004, New York: Churchill Livingstone.

9. Maciocia, G., *Obstretrics & Gynecology in Chinese Medicine.* 1998, New York: Churchhill Livingstone.

10. Rochat De La Vallee, E., *Pregnancy and Gestation in chinese Classical Texts.* 2007: Monkey Press.

11. Mau Kai, C., et al., *Reduced serum testosterone levels in infant boys conceived by intracytoplasmic sperm injection.* J Clin Endocrinol Metab, 2007. **92**(7): p. 2598-603.

12. Ludwig, A., Diedrich, K., Ludwig, M, *The Process of Decision Making in Reproductive Medicine* Semin Reprod Med. 2005;23(4):348-353, 2005. **23**(4): p. 348-353.

13. Lewis, S.E., I. Agbaje, and J. Alvarez, *Sperm DNA tests as useful adjuncts to semen analysis.* Syst Biol Reprod Med, 2008. **54**(3): p. 111-25.

14. Khan, A.e.a., *Cinnamon Improves Glucose and Lipids of People with Type 2 Diabetes.* Diabetes Care, 2003. **26**(12).

15. Dunas, F. *Clinical and Historical Uses of Sexuality: An Oriental Medicine Perspective.* 2012. California: Lotus Institute of Integrative Medicine.

16. Ried, K. and K. Stuart, *Efficacy of Traditional Chinese Herbal Medicine in the management of female infertility: A systematic review.* Complement Ther Clin Pract, 2001. **19**.

17. Lian, F., Z. Sun, and J. Zhang, *Combined therapy of Chinese medicine with in vitro fertilization and embryo transplantation for treatment of polycystic ovarian syndrome.* Zhongguo Zhong Xi Yi Jie He Za Zhi, 2008. **11**: p. 977-980.

18. Wu, R.J. and F.Z. Zhou, *[Effect of yangjing zhongyu decoction on expression of insulin-like growth factor II and its receptor in endometrium of women with unexplained infertility].* Zhongguo Zhong Xi Yi Jie He Za Zhi, 2002. **22**(7): p. 490-3.

19. Battaglia, C., et al., *Adjuvant L-arginine treatment for in-vitro fertilization in poor responder patients.* Human Reproduction, 1999. **14**(7): p. 1690-1697.

20. Tamura, H., et al., *Melatonin and the ovary: physiological and pathophysiological implications.* Fertil Steril, 2009. **92**: p. 328-343.

21. Attaman, J.A.e.a., *Dietary fat and semen quality amongmen attending a fertility clinic.* Human Reproduction, 2012. **0**(0): p. 1-9.

22. Harald Zeisler, C.T., Klaus Mayerhofer, Monir Barrada, Peter Husslein, *Influence of Acupuncture on Duration of Labor.* Gynecol Obstet Invest, 1998. **46**: p. 22-25.

23. Meeker, J.D., et al., *Urinary concentrations of parabens and serum hormone levels, semen quality parameters, and sperm DNA damage.* Environ Health Perspect, 2011. **119**(2): p. 252-7.

24. Meeker, J.D., et al., *Serum Concentrations of Polychlorinated Biphenyls (PCBs) in Relation to in Vitro Fertilization (IVF) Outcomes.* Environ Health Perspect, 2011.

25. Wilson, R.D., et al., *Pre-conceptional vitamin/folic acid supplementation 2007: the use of folic acid in combination with a multivitamin supplement for the prevention of neural tube defects and other congenital anomalies.* J Obstet Gynaecol Can, 2007. **29**(12): p. 1003-26.

26. Guo, J., L.N. Wang, and D. Li, *[Exploring the effects of Chinese medicine in improving uterine endometrial blood flow for increasing the successful rate of in vitro fertilization and embryo transfer].* Zhong Xi Yi Jie He Xue Bao, 2011. **9**(12): p. 1301-6.

27. Kristen, D.e.a., *Intrauterine exposure to mild analgesics is a risk factor for development of male reproductive disorders in human and rat.* Human Reproduction, 2010. **0**(0): p. 1-10.

28. Shamsi, M.B., et al., *DNA integrity and semen quality in men with low seminal antioxidant levels.* Mutat Res, 2009. **665**(1-2): p. 29-36.

29. Cardini, F. and H. Weixin, *Moxibustion for correction of breech presentation: a randomized controlled trial.* JAMA, 1998. **280**(18): p. 1580-4.

30. Liang, L., *Acupuncture & IVF Increaase IVF Success by 40-60%.* 2003, Boulder: Blue Poppy.

31. Betts, D., *The use of acupuncture as a routine pre-birth treatment.* Journal of Chinese Medicine, 2004.

32. Wedenberg, K., B. Moen, and A. Norling, *Acupuncture is better than physiotherapy for low back pain and pelvic pain in pregnancy.* Acta Obstet Gynecol Scand, 2000. **79**: p. 331-335.

33. Sun, F. and J. Yu, *Effect of TCM on plasma beta-endorphin and placental endocrine in threatened abortion.* Zhongguo Zhong Xi Yi Jie He Za Zhi, 1999. **19**(2): p. 87-89.

Appendix-Western Tests & Procedures

Blood Work for Women

- <u>Thyroid Evaluation</u> including: TSH, Free T3, Free T4, Total T4, thyroid antibodies
- <u>Hormone Panel</u> (day 3) should include: P, E2, FSH, LH, Total T, Free T, prolactin, DHEAS, SHBG, AMH
- <u>Fasting Comprehensive Metabolic Panel</u>: CBC, lipid panel, glucose, HbA1c, liver enzymes, etc.
- <u>Vitamin D</u>
- <u>Misc. Testing:</u> genetics, autoimmune markers, inflammatory markers

Blood Work for Men

- <u>Hormone Panel</u>: T, free T, SHBG, LH, FSH, P, prolactin, SHBG
- <u>Fasting Comprehensive Metabolic Panel</u> including: CBC, lipid panel, glucose, HbA1c, liver enzymes, etc.

Procedures for Women

- <u>Pelvic Exam</u>—basic physical exam to ensure that the cervix, uterus and ovaries appear normal and are pain-fee on palpation.
- <u>Ovarian Ultrasound</u>—used to evaluate patients for PCOS, ovarian reserve and to monitor egg development during a drug treatment cycle.
- <u>Sonohysterogram</u>—before the ultrasound, the uterus is filled with a saline solution. Results should show the state of the uterine cavity including polyps, fibroids, abnormal growths or scar tissue.
- <u>Hysterosalpingogram (HSG)</u>—a tube is inserted through the cervix through which a dye is injected. The dye should fill out the uterus and spill through the fallopian tubes. The results should provide information about the uterus and the condition of the fallopian tubes.
- <u>Hysteroscopy</u>—this procedure has both diagnostic and treatment purposes. A camera is used to visualize the uterus and abnormal growths can be removed.
- <u>Laparoscopy</u>—often employed when endometriosis is suspected, this exploratory surgery looks for and removes endometriosis, scar tissue and other abnormal growths.
- <u>Endometrial Biopsy</u>—during the luteal phase, a small piece of endometrial tissue is examined to evaluate uterine lining quality.

Procedures for Men

- <u>Semen Analysis</u>—should include motility, morphology, sperm count, semen quantity and pH, white cells, etc.
- <u>Testicular Biopsy</u>—a piece of the tubules in the testicles is evaluated to determine the quality of sperm production.
- <u>Ultrasound</u>—can be useful in determining if and where blockages are in located in the reproductive tract including the seminal vesicles, the prostate and ejaculatory ducts.

CPSIA information can be obtained at www.ICGtesting.com
Printed in the USA
LVOW10s1935041214

417194LV00020B/1007/P